Learning

GW01424346

in
COMMUNITY
PSYCHIATRIC NURSING

Martin F Ward
RMN, DN(Lond), CertEd(Leeds), RNT, NEBSSDip

Psychiatric Nurse Tutor
Broadland School of Nursing
Norwich

Roy Bishop
RMN, RCNT, RNT, CertEd(Leeds)

Community Psychiatric Nurse Tutor
Broadland School of Nursing
Norwich

HODDER AND STOUGHTON
LONDON   SYDNEY   AUCKLAND   TORONTO

LEARNING TO CARE SERIES

General Editors

JEAN HEATH, MED, BA, SRN, SCM
English National Board Learning Resources Unit, Sheffield

SUSAN E NORMAN, SRN, DNCERT, RNT
Senior Tutor, The Nightingale School, West Lambeth Health Authority

Titles in this series include:

Learning to Care for Elderly People
L THOMAS
Learning to Care in the Community
P TURTON and J ORR
Learning to Care on the Medical Ward
A MATTHEWS
Learnng to Care on the ENT Ward
D STOKES

Learning to Care on the Gynaecology Ward
W SIMONS
Learning to Care for Mentally Handicapped People
V POUNDS
Learning to Care on the PsychiatricWard
M WARD
Learning to Care on the Orthopaedic Ward
D JULIEN

British Library Cataloguing in Publication Data

Ward, Martin F.
    Learning to care in psychiatric nursing.
    – (Learning to care)
    1. Psychiatric nursing – Great Britain
    I. Title   II. Bishop, Roy   III. Series
    610.73'68'0941   RC440

ISBN 0 340 39918 X

First published 1986

Typeset in 10/11 pt Trump Mediaeval by Rowland Phototypesetting Ltd, Bury St Edmunds, Suffolk

Printed in Great Britain for Hodder and Stoughton Educational, a division of Hodder and Stoughton Ltd, Mill Road, Dunton Green, Sevenoaks, Kent TN13 2YD, by Richard Clay (The Chaucer Press) Ltd, Bungay, Suffolk

EDITORS' FOREWORD

In most professions there is a traditional gulf between theory and its practice, and nursing is no exception. The gulf is perpetuated when theory is taught in a theoretical setting and practice is taught by the practitioner.

This inherent gulf has to be bridged by students of nursing, and publication of this series is an attempt to aid such bridge building.

It aims to help relate theory and practice in a meaningful way whilst underlining the importance of the person being cared for.

It aims to introduce students of nursing to some of the more common problems found in each new area of experience in which they will be asked to work.

It aims to de-mystify some of the technical language they will hear, putting it in context, giving it meaning and enabling understanding.

PREFACE

If you open any dictionary and look for the word 'community', you will be surprised at the number of different ways there are of saying, 'a group of people living in the same locality'. You will find such phrases as common fellowship and common interests, but you will find nothing that suggests the real fabric of a community where each member has a role to play, and a price to pay should he fail to do so.

For one in ten of the population of the UK, the price so often paid is that of mental illness. An early 16th century proverb reads, 'Everyman is the architect of his own design', interesting but not necessarily true. Very often the community itself may be responsible in part for causing psychiatric problems to develop and to a degree the community psychiatric nurse (CPN) has a responsibility to help redress that balance. People who have suffered the effects of mental illness need special support, guidance and reassurance if they are to lead satisfying and purposeful lives. That help will come from many quarters, but within the community none is more specialised than the CPN.

This book, designed basically for nurse learners, does not try to identify completely the role of the CPN but rather the skills she might use and the situations in which she might use them. Helping an individual to function simply as a member of a community requires the co-operation of many people so the book also considers how the CPN fits into the support team for the care of the mentally ill in modern society.

CONTENTS

Introduction

If you are allocated to a particular type of ward as part of your training you are no doubt interested in the characteristics of that ward. Where is it? What type of ward is it? How is it organised? What are the patients and staff like? The answers to these questions help you to build up your personal confidence and form an initial framework of ideas about the place in which you are going to work and learn. They may also, of course, contribute to your negative preconceptions about the ward, and so make the allocation one to be approached with trepidation. Nevertheless it is always worth examining the construct of the ward and its members.

The community allocation during psychiatric nurse education provokes negative feelings in some and positive feelings in others; very few students feel neutral about what is seen as a different working environment. The same questions can be asked about the community as can be asked about a ward. It may be useful at this point to quote a definition of the term 'community' as it is used by sociologists:

> A community is a human group living within a limited and defined geographical area in which they carry out most of their day to day activities. (Jones & Jones 1975)

We can see from this definition that we are talking about a smaller group than when we use the term 'society'. Although a number of communities comprise a whole society, it is important not to confuse the two concepts. In nursing terms, the ward can be seen as a community which is part of the whole hospital and if we stay with the Jones definition it is easy to see that the continuing care ward is as much a community in itself as is a village, town or city. In the majority of continuing care wards, day to day life is dictated by routines and by the needs of both patients and staff in order to allow the ward community to function as a cohesive group. Meal times are usually fixed and various activities follow a timed programme which may change only slightly from year to year. The communities outside the hospital often function in much the same way and are often just as limiting as life within the continuing care ward. Just think how much your life is governed by the community in which you live: are, for instance, meal times entirely your own choice? Can you stay in bed as long as you want?

Your community allocation requires of you an understanding of communal life, its pressures, pains and pleasures, but most of all an appreciation that the skills of a psychiatric nurse are as relevant and as appropriate here as they are in traditional hospital work. The setting in which those skills are used may be different but the people who benefit from them are members of a community wherever they are staying.

The Concept of Community

It is possible to live in total isolation from other people, but few choose to do so and modern society makes such a choice increasingly unlikely. Our relationships with others are very important to us and can often be seen as the main cohesive element in our community lives. Note how any threat to the

Continuing care In the sense in which the word is used here, we refer to the care of the long term resident of the psychiatric hospital and emphasise the fact that this care is continuing rather than circumscribed as it often is in the case of a short stay (acute) patient.

Community networks – a network is an inter-relationship between people, organisations and situations. In a community sense it could include family, friends, work, church or even the local pub.

continuance of community networks causes unrest, insecurity and even aggression, especially in those who place high value on their relationships with others. It is probably in response to this type of threat that various community developments have taken place during recent years. Community oriented approaches have become predominant in health and social services, education and policing. However, these provisions on the one hand can be seen as forces which dictate our style of life and our behaviour toward one another. The recipients of psychiatric nursing in the community outside the hospital are subject to the same influences as those people who provide that care, but it is difficult to see that relationship in the same way within the ward community. The setting in which community psychiatric nursing skills are used is the one in which most of us live and it seems appropriate at this point to look at how our behaviour influences, and is influenced by, the community in which we live.

Interactional indicates person to person communications in everyday life, including such personal skills as being assertive without being aggressive, and coping with conversation.
Socially defined – some behaviour is said to be 'natural' and not the consequence of social organisation. Behaviour that is socially defined is agreed generally to be the product of contact between individuals and amounts to a standard or norm.

Behaviour in the Community

If a person is unable to perform everyday personal and interactional tasks in a way which his community regards as normal or acceptable he may find other people assume there is something wrong with him: he may feel there is something wrong himself. What is seen as normal behaviour is to a great extent socially defined, for the norm in one community may well be unacceptable in another. Take for instance the long term resident of a psychiatric hospital who for years has collected cigarette ends from various ash trays and feels no discomfort in doing so within the hospital community. If he performs the same activity in a public place, those who see him do it are likely to assume his behaviour to be socially unacceptable and feel there is something wrong with him. The disapproving reaction shown to such a person can be a source of confusion to him and may influence many of his other everyday activities and his feeling towards himself. Such people may become socially isolated and find great difficulty understanding the interactional technicalities of the community in which they live.

So, it seems that to live comfortably in any community we must learn the rules and abide by them. Mental disorders may deprive people of their ability to conform to social norms by virtue of their tendency to produce behaviour and feelings which the community regards as unacceptable or inappropriate. Conversely, it could be said that the failure to master social and personal skills can make a person liable to mental disorder. One way or the other, behaviour in a community setting is the social yardstick by which we are all measured. If our behaviour leads to our being seen by a doctor, the term 'mental illness' may be used to answer the question, 'What is wrong with you?' If we find ourselves in conflict with the laws of the community, our behaviour may result in our being labelled as criminal. This conflict in explanation of behaviour has led to much debate, particularly the 'mad or bad' argument. If a member of the community breaks the rules, we often find ourselves asking, 'How could he do this thing?' If the behaviour is particularly upsetting to a large number of people, there is a greater tendency to describe the offender as abnormal and can lead to imprisonment or compulsory admission to a psychiatric hospital. In order to protect itself, the community defines normality and abnormality.

We can see how various influences bring pressure on us to behave in particular ways, but life is not that pessimistic really. Occasionally we kick back at these pressures in order to assert our individuality.

Some of the influences on the individual which constrain him to conform to normality

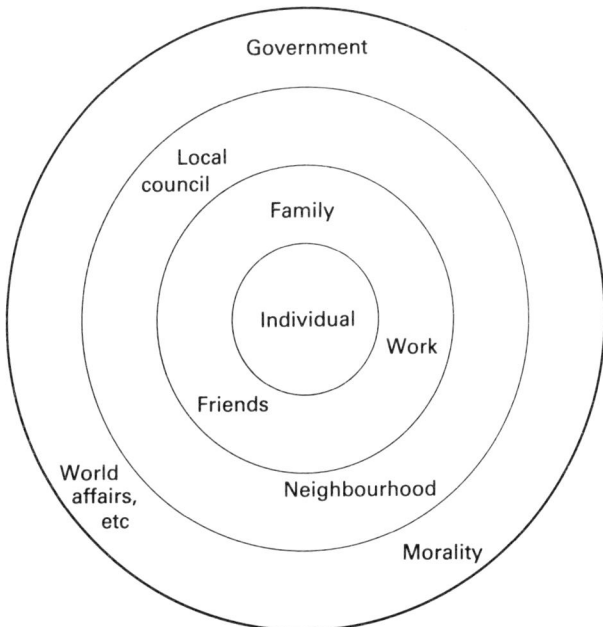

Not all those individuals suffering mental disorders are segregated from the community at large. In fact, most are treated in the community and never come into contact with hospital in-patient care. Thomas (1983), for example, found only 16 per cent of 300 referrals to a psychiatric liaison service in Leicester required admission to hospital. The table on p. 6 illustrates similar findings in relation to the elderly and mental disorder. Most of us can think of people within our own communities who are generally regarded as eccentric or odd but who do not pose any threat to our social stability or personal safety. Indeed there are signs that people are becoming more tolerant of mental upsets and even admit to feeling depressed or anxious themselves, thus developing some degree of empathy with those who previously may have been feared and segregated.

Empathy is the ability to see things from the viewpoint of the other person rather than purely from our own experience. It is not the same as sympathy since that feeling reflects *our own* view.

Estimated total prevalence rates for the main psychiatric disorders per 1000 population aged 65 years and over

Main disorder	Prevalence per 1000 aged 65+ years	Ratio of patients living at home vs living in institutions
Severe brain syndromes	56	6:1
Mild brain syndromes	57	10:1
Manic depressive disorder	14	18:1
Schizophrenia (excluding long stay mental hospital patients)	11	9:1
Neurotic and personality states	125	51:1
All disorders	263	14:1

It is into this improved atmosphere that the community psychiatric nurse is being thrust at the same time that many long-stay residents of psychiatric hospitals are leaving the protection of their institution. Unusual behaviour in the community may or may not become more apparent due to these two major shifts. Whatever happens, the skills of psychiatric nursing need to be developed for use away from the confines of the traditional mental hospital. The outmoded custodial approach is replaced by a more positive and hopeful attempt to enable vulnerable or difficult people to live more effectively within the community at minimum risk to themselves or others.

Concepts of Care: Community or Hospital?

Is everything about the large psychiatric hospital bad? Is the new community approach the best development ever to have taken place in the care of the mentally disordered? These questions may well appear extreme as they are poles apart but unless we ask them we may miss the essential features of each care philosophy. To dismiss the hospital without looking for its virtues or to accept community care without acknowledging its failings would not do justice to either system.

The large mental hospital, so familiar in the British countryside, developed in response to many social and economic circumstances. Private 'madhouses' made good money for those who ran them and many a rich inheritance has a certified lunatic in its past. The poor who became mentally unwell certainly could not afford the dubious luxury of private attention and, for the most part, lived in workhouses or wandered the city streets and country lanes. The wandering insane caused fear, embarrassment and guilt to the community and to some extent it was the public outcry which led to the development of institutions to afford protection for both parties. So it seems that mental hospitals run by the state came into being partly because the mentally disordered were poorly treated by the community . . . an important point to note when examining the concept of care in the community today.

An institution is more than bricks and mortar; it has a social meaning which applies to an organisation with rules and social structure.

Huge insular monuments to an era of moral condemnation, the mental hospitals proved to be rigid, authoritarian and powerful. They provided sanctuary for the mentally disordered and protection for the community but little in the way of successful treatment. Also, to enter a mental hospital meant stigmatisation and small chance of rejoining the community under the same circumstances as you left it. The institutions themselves became more important than the patients they were there to help. The rigid system proved a fertile ground on which to plant professional status, and to some extent we in the profession have reaped the harvest of this, whether we want it or not. Psychiatric nurse education and practice first developed in the large mental hospitals and it is that heritage which makes the transfer of skills to a less formal community setting difficult to achieve.

In hospital the patient becomes the recipient of the nurse's care and if there is no improvement, the nurse has the strength of the institution and the power of her status to protect her. She can go home when off duty knowing that someone else is providing care in her absence and the overall passivity of the patient is maintained. The hospital is so big and the staff so important that they may overshadow the importance of the care of the patient. If you were admitted to your local general hospital tonight suffering from severe pain and you found yourself still there, with your pain, in twenty years' time, you could be justified in asking for another opinion as to your treatment. It can be said that developments in social psychiatry and nursing are a response to the failure of the large hospital system.

However, there may always be a need for emergency, short term, in-patient care in the treatment of mental disorder and some people may always need the security and protection of a specialised unit. Neither of these facilities needs to be huge in size or remote in location; they should meet the needs of the local community, and help *within* the community should be the major strategy. Community care may never entirely replace hospital care but it is important to be aware of the advantages and disadvantages of both. Helping the mentally disordered in their own homes and localities can help reduce the stigma of illness and allow the individual to maintain independence and self respect. Without the power of the institution to cling to, the nurse can more easily develop skills which are person oriented and not dependent on the necessary rules of a large mental hospital. Both nurses and patients are more exposed without the security of the hospital but that is the challenge we face as people *and* as nurses; that certainly is the excitement of community psychiatric nursing.

Advantages and disadvantages of care strategies

Institutional care	
Advantages	**Disadvantages**
Concentration of resources	Isolation from community
Safety and protection	Institutionalism
Therapeutic environment can be produced	Authoritarian atmosphere may develop
24 hr cover available	Patient label usually applied
	Reduced personal status
	Often housed in unsuitable and outdated buildings

Community care	
Advantages	**Disadvantages**
Retention of social contacts	Lack of resources for the discharged old long stay group
Less stigma	Presence of mentally ill in the community may worsen prejudices
Patient label can be avoided	
Emphasis on people not buildings	
Help provided in personal environment	Vulnerable people difficult to protect from the unscrupulous
Less formality in nurse–client relationship	

TEST YOURSELF	1 How does the community define who is ill and who is well? 2 What are the advantages and disadvantages of community psychiatric care?

3   What sort of facilities are available in your area for: in-patient psychiatric care? out-patient psychiatric care?

FURTHER READING

BUTTERWORTH, C. A. & SKIDMORE, D. 1981. *Caring for the Mentally Ill in the Community.* Beckenham: Croom Helm.

CARR, P. J., BUTTERWORTH, C. A. & HODGES, B. E. 1979. *Community Psychiatric Nursing.* Edinburgh: Churchill Livingstone.

HEMSI, L. 1980. Psychogeriatric Care in the Community. *Health Trends,* **12**:25–9.

JONES, R. K. & JONES, P. A. 1975. *Sociology in Medicine.* Sevenoaks: Hodder and Stoughton.

MANGEN, S. 1982. *Sociology and Mental Health.* Edinburgh: Churchill Livingstone.

MILES, A. 1981. *The Mentally Ill in Contemporary Society.* Oxford: Martin Robertson.

MIND. 1983. *Care in the Community: Keeping it local.* Report of Mind's 1983 annual conference. London.

THOMAS, C. 1983. Referrals to a British Liaison Psychiatric Service. *Health Trends,* **15**:61–4.

2 Organisation of Community Psychiatric Nursing Services

Management and Organisation

During psychiatric nurse training, the community experience usually represents only one module in the whole course. Also, it is often presented after the student has been exposed to a great deal of ward based work, so it is not surprising that many find adaptation to the new environment quite difficult. After experiencing the comparatively rigid approach to such matters as working hours, uniforms, work rate and hierarchy-dictated professional relationships, the less supervised day spent by the CPN is hard to adapt to. Indeed many community psychiatric nurses themselves seem to be quite critical of the way their job is viewed by the hospital nurse, and in particular by hospital based nurse managers.

Skidmore and Friend (1983) found CPNs to be generally dissatisfied with a number of management relationship problems, particularly if community teams were managed by those without community experience. Many expressed the wish to be managed by an experienced CPN with a small caseload of his or her own.

So how is the average CPN team organised and managed? Although this may seem a simple enough question, it becomes more complicated on closer examination.

Firstly, there appears to be no such 'animal' as an average CPN team. Surveys have revealed an enormous range of working practices and management styles. Some teams are managed by a senior nurse who also has responsibilities for a number of hospital wards, whilst others have a team manager who is solely employed for that purpose.

Secondly, because community care is a relatively young concept, there is little evidence to point to the most favourable and efficient manner of organising the nursing component of the overall multi-disciplinary approach it represents.

A further complication is the implementation of the Griffiths report on health service management, in which senior managers from industry and commerce have been recruited by many authorities. Although these managers in the main possess a high degree of management expertise, they do not necessarily possess much knowledge about, nor emphasise, the quality of care. This is further complicated by the difficulty of defining what is meant by 'quality of care'. The problem for community psychiatric nursing seems to be that many of the new managers feel that only one community nurse manager is required for all the nursing specialists. Hence, some community psychiatric nursing teams are managed by people with no psychiatric nursing experience at all. However, despite this, many teams have developed an organised and forward looking approach to providing a service for the mentally disordered person in the community, and the learner allocated to this experience has a wonderful opportunity to be involved in the early stages of growth in a new service.

In order to examine these varied systems, it is helpful to ask the following questions:

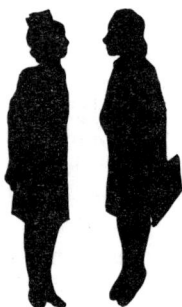

1 To whom is the CPN responsible?
2 Where does the CPN work from?
3 How are patients referred to the CPN?

1 *Lines of responsibility*
In any hierarchical management relationship, there are a number of possible alternatives of responsibility, each with its own advantages and disadvantages. However, the CPN works at charge nurse level most often and is responsible to a senior nurse who is in turn responsible to a senior or divisional nurse manager. Some teams have staff nurses and enrolled nurses, but those CPNs who make up the largest number nationally are of charge nurse 2 grade. A very good account of the possible management relationship organisation is given by Carr *et al.* (1979).

2 *Operational bases*
The vast majority of CPNs still work from the psychiatric hospital, but this number has been declining over recent years in favour of using health centres/GP practices. An increasing number of CPNs are based in such areas as community health centres, day centres for the elderly, various community bases and rehabilitation centres. Due to the increasing drive toward providing locally based community care groups, it is probable that this growth in community based CPNs will continue and the number of hospital based CPNs will decline further. It is an interesting exercise to look at these developments within the CPN team to which you are attached.

3 *Referral systems*
Because of the large number of CPNs still based in hospital, psychiatrists tend to be the main source of referral; indeed most CPNs are still allocated to particular consultants and referrals originate from that association. Many teams, however, have developed an 'open referral' system in which anyone (district

nurses, social services, relatives and the patients themselves) has access. An increasing number of referrals come from GPs because a growing number of CPNs are attached to health centres and GP surgeries.

Examples of CPN Service Organisation

In order to present an indication of how a CPN service might be properly organised, two examples are given. Although the general principles are similar in both cases, one major difference between them is that in service 'A' the CPNs are formed into teams serving specific geographical areas whilst in service 'B' the addition of the CPN specialty represents a further modification.

Service A: CPN Service Organisation

Community senior nurse (team leader)

Area 1	Area 2	Area 3	Area 4
CPN CPN	CPN CPN	CPN CPN	CPN CPN
Based in psychiatric hospital	Health centre based	Health centre based	Based in community health centre

Service B: CPN Service Organisation using clinical specialties

Community senior nurse (team leader)

Team 1	Team 2	Team 3	Team 4
CPN CPN	CPN CPN	CPN CPN	CPN CPN
Care of the elderly mentally ill	Care of drug, alcohol and solvent abusers	Responsibility for rehabilitation	Care of the acute mentally ill

In both services there are the same number of team leaders and CPNs but service 'A' staff can work generically, whereas service 'B' staff would specialise in their work irrespective of the area from which the referral originates.

Generically is used here to indicate that community psychiatric nursing is provided for any person referred within the area covered by the CPN.

There are many facets to the debate concerning area allocation or CPN specialisation, and some services manage to practise both.

Explanatory note: where CPNs do specialise, the largest group seem to concentrate on the care of the elderly. The more specialist the work becomes, the fewer CPNs work in it. For example, only a very small number of CPNs specialise in such areas as family therapy, behaviour therapy or child adolescent work; a CPN team leader might see such a specialist as a luxury not to be afforded in spite of the history of success which is associated with nurses working in these specialties. For further discussion on the development of specialty functions for CPNs see Chapter 9 where we look at the future of community psychiatric nursing.

Management and organisation of CPN services are continually evolving. Experience, coupled with the lively communication between CPNs from various parts of the country which is generally afforded through such forums as conferences, study days and the Community Psychiatric Nurses' Association, will undoubtedly lead to the development of more established management practices. The high standard of the CPNs emerging from the English National Board course in community psychiatric nursing should also lead to a more informed approach to service organisation.

Professional Relationships

CPNs are rapidly establishing themselves as important members of the community care multi-disciplinary team. It is important here to briefly mention the relationships between those people who are involved in the care of the mentally disordered in the community.

1 *Primary Health Care Team*
Primary health care can be defined as the provision of services at the point of first contact, such as when the person seeks assistance from

a General Practitioner. This does not mean, however, that the responsibility of those working in primary health begins with the ill person; there is also a preventative aspect to this service. The primary health care team is not a new concept and some of its members have been practising in this area for many years. Recently the size of these teams has increased to meet the need identified over years of experience but it could be said that originally the general practitioner and the district nurse comprised the whole team.

Nowadays, the team consists of a care team of doctors, nurses, health visitors, social workers and medical secretaries with other health care professionals making up the wider team (Bailey 1981). The nursing membership usually consists of the health visitor, the midwife, the district nurse and the practice nurse.

It is in this team that the CPN is rapidly making an increasing contribution. With the growth of community care for the mentally disordered and the recognition of the importance of mental health education, the need to attach psychiatric nurses to health centre based teams has been established. As we saw earlier in this chapter, an increasing number of CPNs are moving away from the hospital setting and joining the primary health care teams in the community.

Explanatory note: the professional relationship between the established primary health care team members and the CPN is in a state of evolution, and in many ways the CPNs joining the team are pioneers for the psychiatric nursing of the mentally ill within the community. The CPN must be able to establish professional working relationships with other team members, and demonstrate the wide range of services the psychiatric nurse can contribute to the team as a whole.

2 *Hospital services*
It would be a mistake to imagine that the community psychiatric nurse could work in

total isolation from the psychiatric in-patient service and the need for close liaison between hospital and community nursing care is widely accepted.

The CPN must have contact with the local in-patient facility in order to receive referrals and to follow up those people who have had to be admitted in spite of community care provision. The CPN is therefore involved with admission and discharge referrals.

Admission referrals These would stem either from members of an existing case load when community care fails to maintain the individual's mental health, or from direct referral to the CPN from other members of the primary health care team. In both cases, the necessity for the CPN to maintain a personal link with the individual whilst in hospital is

The CPN's involvement in admission and discharge referrals

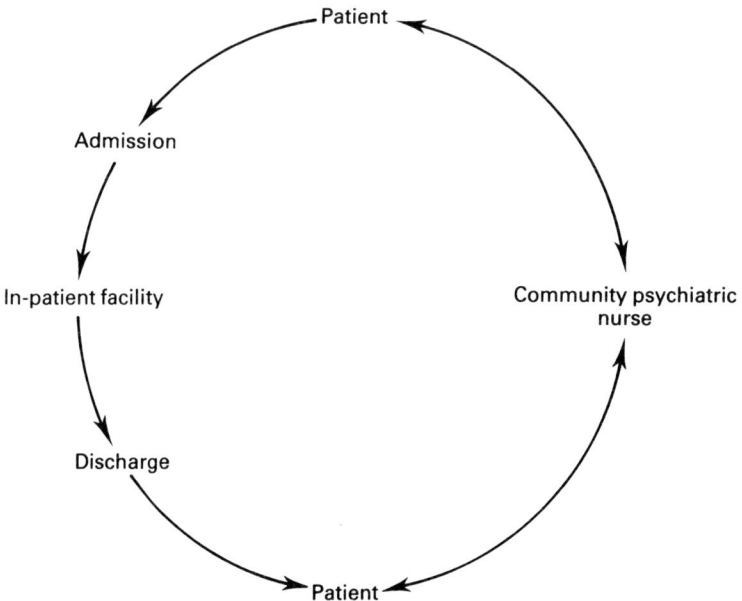

essential. It enables the CPN to monitor the effects of treatment on her patient and give the patient a sense of being cared about by the CPN – which is an essential element of care when he eventually returns to the community once again.

Discharge referrals Individuals being discharged from hospital will almost always need the support, guidance and monitoring that the CPN is able to provide. Of course, each case will differ, but it is important that links are established or monitored prior to the person being discharged. In this way, both parties can get to know each other and begin to formulate a pattern of care that will take over once the 'cotton wool environment' of in-patient facilities has been left behind.

'Cotton wool environment' is often used to describe in-patient psychiatric care where patients may be shielded from the harshness of everyday problems and decision making.

3 *Voluntary organisations*

It is time to say that without the voluntary organisations, the statutory bodies would be unable to cope with the pressure of work necessary to maintain the many thousands of people who live in the community suffering the effects of psychiatric problems. These organisations vary in size and responsibility, ranging from small self help groups dealing with the problems of anorexia, alcohol abuse and bereavement, to the major national organisations and trusts such as MIND and the Richmond Fellowship. Some have religious affiliations while others are bonded only by the determination of those who organise them to live as normal and satisfying a life as possible. Although some of these groups offer help to people within hospital, most of their energy is directed towards community care, support and guidance. The CPN's involvement with these organisations often forms that very important link which maintains care continuity.

The CPN's knowledge of how the various voluntary groups work and for whom may enable her to use their specialist help in a particular individual's care programme. By so doing she can probably increase the time available to her for seeing other patients whilst ensuring a more individualised and pertinent form of care for certain members of her case load.

The voluntary organisations receive reciprocal support from the CPNs who also refer to them people who will benefit from their help. In this way, the groups and the CPN complement each other to provide care specifically orientated towards the needs of the individual and their relatives and friends, rather than simple blanket care.

Concluding Remarks

The CPN cannot function effectively if she isolates herself and tries to provide care for her patients based solely on her own skills. She must form and maintain good channels of communication with all other interested parties, so that she becomes the central co-ordinator in the care network. She must identify for herself what is available, how it can be utilised and what it will take in both financial and human terms to use it for the benefit of her patients. In return, she can offer other health professionals an insight into the patient's community existence. The increase in effectiveness consistent with such relationships will inevitably be passed onto the patient.

TEST YOURSELF

1 In the text two approaches to the organisation of CPN services are discussed. What are the advantages and disadvantages of these structures?
2 How does the CPN fit into the established primary health care team?
3 If CPNs are based in the community rather

than in hospitals, how might this affect their work practice in relation to referrals, response to care, and individual role?

FURTHER READING

BALY, M. E. (ed) 1984. *A New Approach to District Nursing*. London: Heinemann Medical Books Ltd.

BYRNE, T. & PADFIELD, C. F. 1985. *Social Services*. London: Heinemann.

COMMUNITY PSYCHIATRIC NURSES' ASSOCIATION. 1985. *The 1985 CPNA National Survey*. Update. Bristol: CPNA.

DAVIES, J. B. 1983. *Community Health, Preventative Medicine and Social Services*. Eastbourne: Baillière Tindall.

DICKINSON, P. 1984. The CPN in Primary Health Care. *Community Psychiatric Nursing Journal*, **4**(5):6–10.

REED, J. & LOMAS, G. (ed) 1984. *Psychiatric Services in the Community: Developments and Innovations*. Beckenham: Croom Helm.

WILLIAMSON, F., LITTLE, M. & LINDSAY, W. 1981. The Community Psychiatric Nursing Services Compared. *Nursing Times*, **77**(27):105–7.

WING, J. K. & OLSEN, R. 1979. *Community Care for the Mentally Disabled*. Oxford: Oxford University Press.

3 The Skills of Anxiety Management

Anxiety is a state of emotional and physical arousal which is characterised by feelings of apprehension and fear and is usually accompanied by physical responses such as sweating, tremor and nausea.

Anxiety is a normal emotion. Far from being a mental disorder, it is a positive state which occurs so that we can function efficiently in response to many situations. For example, when taking an important examination a student needs to be a little anxious in order to stimulate his performance to a level which tests his ability to recall and apply what he has learnt. If he remains too calm and relaxed, he is likely to have difficulty in responding to the demands of the situation.

This is illustrated by the 'Yerkes–Dodson Law' which states that low levels and high levels of emotional arousal are accompanied by low levels of performance, whereas a medium level of arousal produces good performance. In other words, moderate levels of anxiety can enable the person to perform at an optimum level but under or over stimulation will lower performance. (See figure on next page.)

However, if anxiety becomes the predominant emotional state in a person for no particular reason, or in response to circumstances or objects which are not normally anxiety provoking, then a problem can be said to exist. In these situations it seems that the person has a decreased ability to control anxiety and the emotional state appears to be controlling him. It is not unusual for the person to suffer anxiety to such a degree that it becomes terror and leads to panic. The inability to control anxiety usually leads to the request for help. The diagnosis will be of an anxiety state if it occurs in a general way, or of phobic anxiety if it is

Yerkes–Dodson's Law

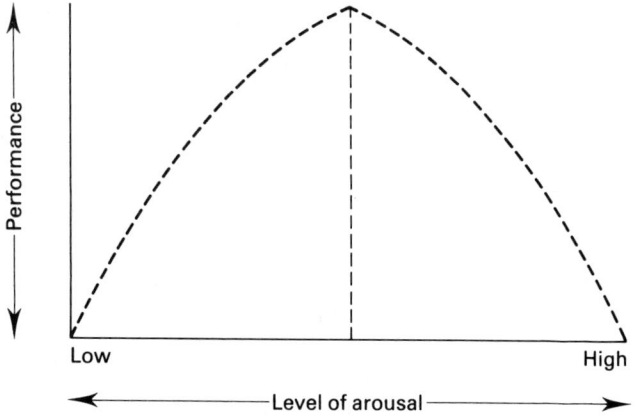

related to a specific situation or object.

The community psychiatric nurse frequently encounters the anxious person and it is important that she has the necessary skills, knowledge and attitudes to help, both on a one to one basis and within a group. Some anxious people may derive sufficient benefit from the regular reassuring attention of a CPN whilst others may respond better to structured meetings with groups of fellow sufferers organised by the CPN at the local health centre.

Knowledge and attitudes developed during basic RMN training are as applicable in community psychiatric work as they are in hospital practice. It is the use of particular skills which can extend the nurse's function to show a difference between hospital and community psychiatric care of anxious people.

Explanatory note: it is worth pointing out at this time that many members of the health care team spend very long periods of training to develop specific therapeutic skills which are often beyond the scope and capabilities of the basically trained psychiatric nurse. For the CPN to offer herself as a therapist, it is essential for her to undergo proper training in whatever therapy she wishes to use.

This does not debar the CPN from practising some forms of help for the anxious person and there are two particular areas where she can be of use, with supervision and advice from an experienced person. These two areas are generally regarded as constituting what many CPNs refer to as anxiety management techniques:

1   Relaxation therapy.
2   Desensitisation.

Relaxation Therapy

This therapy is an ideal technique for the CPN to develop for use either in the patient's home or in a group at the local health centre.

The basis of relaxation therapy is the knowledge that the ability to relax is a natural one and that most people are able to relax without really having to try. Those who find difficulty in controlling anxiety levels usually are unable to relax and so some help in developing their natural ability can be very useful if they can apply it at crucial times. For example, being able to employ relaxation skills during a period which could provoke anxiety may bring some idea of how to gain control over the situation.

It is important that the technique is learned in such a way that it can be used in everyday situations which may produce stress for the individual. It is not going to be any good to learn a technique which always requires a bed, a darkened room and two free hours. Relaxation in those conditions is important and would probably help if the circumstances were right, but it is more important to learn the method in such a way that it can be practised under pressure, at work, when shopping or in the pub.

This means that two phases of relaxation should be taught to the patient. The first, deep

Stress is a demand on energy produced by the strain of coping with a threatening or difficult situation, usually resulting in a feeling of fatigue.

relaxation, is best learned in a warm, comfortable and safe environment while the second, tension control, can be a development used in virtually any situation.

Explanatory note: deep relaxation involves following a set pattern of progressive muscular tensing and relaxing. For example, clenching the fist and then relaxing it allows the person to experience the feeling of immense difference between relaxation and tension. This gradually progresses until as many muscle groups as possible have been tensed and relaxed.

There are many pre-recorded audio tapes available which systematically progress through a routine using a soft reassuring voice. The CPN can use these tapes rather than recite the routine herself, if she wishes. Regular use of this technique can help the anxious person realise that tension control is contained within himself and the ability to cope and control anxiety is a natural ability which can be developed. Once the person is able to relax in the safe, warm and secure environment and has developed the knowledge of self control, the technique can be refined and adjusted to be of use in controlling tension in everyday situations anywhere. It is not the intention to explain these techniques in detail at this point since the care study following this first part of the chapter will illustrate them in practice.

Desensitisation

This technique is useful when, as the name implies, a person has become sensitive to an object or situation to such a degree that this sensitivity interferes with his ability to carry on normally in life to his own or other people's satisfaction. A psychologist would refer to this as a phobia. Since it is thought that most phobias are learned responses, the priority in treatment is usually to help the person 'unlearn' or to become 'densensitised'.

Desensitisation usually begins with the person learning relaxation techniques to enable him to relax, almost on demand. Following this, he may be gradually introduced to the object or situation which brings about anxiety for him, and encouraged to use the relaxation skills while in the fear state.

This technique, while being relatively straightforward to use, does require considerable help from the therapist and it would be unwise for the CPN to attempt to use it without the advice of a psychologist or psychiatrist. Ideally one CPN could attend a course of training in behaviour therapy and could then help other CPNs to develop these skills for use with their patients.

The second half of this chapter gives an example of both techniques actually being used by a community psychiatric nurse in the case of a lady who has developed a fear which has become associated with a specific object/situation. Phobias, as these states are called, are often very suitable for a combination of relaxation and desensitisation treatments.

Behaviour therapy involves therapeutic techniques based on the theory that what people actually do is the most important thing to change, as opposed to what they think has motivated them.

Phobia is a morbid state of irrational fear exhibited whenever the sufferer is in contact with a particular object or situation which is normally harmless. Where possible, he avoids the cause of fear and 'panic attacks' may occur if this is not possible.

Jill who has phobic anxiety

HISTORY

Phobic reaction is the behaviour exhibited by an individual in response to a phobia, or irrational fear.

Jill was referred directly to the community psychiatric nurse from her own GP because she was complaining of behaviour consistent with a phobic reaction. She appeared to have a dread of being in open spaces, such as large shops, parks, gardens, or just the High Street. She had only managed to get to the doctor's surgery because her mother had promised to stay with her throughout the journey and the consultation. It came to light that she had not been able to get Jill out of the house for several days prior to the appointment and on the doctor's advice had not mentioned either the time or date of the appointment in case this aroused more anxiety. Jill was given two choices by the doctor:

1 Drugs which would help her combat the effects of anxiety and hopefully make her feel more relaxed when confronted by her phobic situations.

2 Or referral to the community psychiatric nurse for a programme of controlled relaxation and desensitisation.

Anxiolytic medication is drugs used to combat anxiety such as Valium (diazepam), Librium (chlordiazepoxide).

She chose a combination of both. Anxiolytic medication was prescribed to help her cope with the anxiety until the programme began, the dosage gradually being reduced as the programme helped her cope more effectively on her own.

Explanatory note: direct referral from a doctor to a community psychiatric nurse attached to a health centre or community practice is often the best method of using specialist skills associated with psychiatric training. The doctor would thus be aware of any particular therapy or skill that the nurse has to offer; in the case of desensitisation the nurse may well have attended a behaviour therapy course. This form of medical/nursing integration enables the nurse to exercise her autonomous role whilst releasing the doctor to spend more time with other patients. This type of referral is particularly suitable for the nurse because it requires the establishment of a good patient–nurse relationship and then quite a considerable education programme before eventually leading to patient independence. Models of nursing which see the nurse as a care agent promoting patient competence are complementary to this form of skills care. Because the programme needs to involve the patient's relatives, the fact that it will take place within the family home rather than a clinic or out-patient department is also of great importance.

FIRST VISIT

The nurse's introductory visit was very much a low key affair designed to allow both parties to get to know each other as well as possible. They discussed the problems surrounding

Jill's agoraphobia, its presentation and general effects upon her behaviour. Next they considered what the programme of care was intended to do. The nurse explained that she would visit Jill in her home twice weekly for the next few weeks, gradually reducing the time spent, and then the frequency of the visits until Jill was able to cope more effectively on her own. At that time, the care programme would be reviewed once again to see both what was still required for Jill's peace of mind, and what the nurse was in a position to offer. The necessity to involve Jill's mother in the programme, certainly during the initial stages, was stressed and Jill readily agreed to this.

The method of teaching relaxation was discussed in some depth and it was explained that once Jill had begun to master the technique then the process of desensitisation would begin. She was to continue with her medication until she felt more capable of coping without it at which time the situation would be reviewed by both the nurse and the doctor.

So that Jill could receive something positive from this first visit, the nurse left a relaxation cassette tape for her simply to listen to. She also asked her to make a list of those things or situations which seemed to cause the most anxiety, explaining that at her next visit they would place these items in order of anxiety provocation. The date of the next visit was arranged and the nurse left Jill to consider her list.

ASSESSMENT at introductory visit

This first visit with Jill indicated the amount of time that would be required to counter the effects of anxiety through relaxation therapy. The length of time had to be established at the beginning so that Jill could have a personal contract to which she would be obliged to commit herself. In this way she began to take some responsibility for her care programme and gained some initial confidence in the therapy situation.

The nurse was also able to establish the future level of her own input in relation to Jill's problem. Each individual visited by the nurse would require the general programme to be tailored specifically for them, taking into consideration such factors as the severity of the condition, their willingness to undertake the care programme, the support of others and the actual response to the nurse. In Jill's case the nurse had discovered that this pattern of behaviour was relatively new and concluded that, as a consequence, it might be possible to overcome it equally as quickly. This was important as the more deep seated the behaviour becomes, the more difficult it is to change it. No attempt was made at this point to establish why she was behaving as she was.

FIRST THERAPY VISIT

Two days later when the nurse visited, Jill had both listened to the tape and begun to carry out the instructions on it despite not having been asked to do so. This was a good sign because it indicated a desire to get involved. Secondly, she had also made out her list which she and the nurse proceeded to place in a hierarchy of anxiety provocation. To do this, the nurse simply asked Jill to grade each item with a number, 1 for that evoking the most anxiety and 10 for that which generated the least. This completed hierarchy would form the basis for the desensitisation programme. This range of intensity enabled the nurse to plot the anxiety level for each item and would act as a baseline for future assessment of Jill's progress.

The nurse next suggested that the relaxation programme should begin.

Hierarchy of problems for Jill

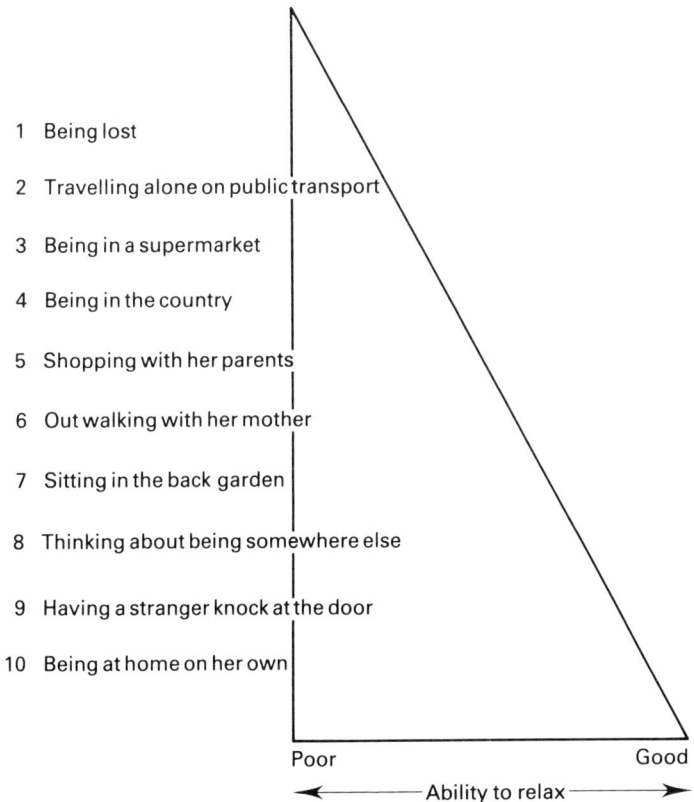

1 Being lost

2 Travelling alone on public transport

3 Being in a supermarket

4 Being in the country

5 Shopping with her parents

6 Out walking with her mother

7 Sitting in the back garden

8 Thinking about being somewhere else

9 Having a stranger knock at the door

10 Being at home on her own

Poor   Good

◄──────── Ability to relax ────────►

Explanatory note: before the process of desensitisation
can begin, the patient must learn how to control the
physical response to anxiety. In this way she is able to
make her body do as she wishes, rather than allowing
it to control her. In therapy, if a relaxing feeling can be
produced during an anxiety provoking situation, anxiety
itself can ultimately be brought under control.

Jill's mother was present at this first therapy
session as the nurse needed to teach both of
them how the programme worked. In this way,
Mother would take responsibility for over-
seeing the required homework set by the

nurse, ensuring that continuity was maintained between visits.

Relaxation Techniques

The tape lasted for approximately 20 minutes. All Jill needed to do was to follow the instructions on the tape, whilst Mother watched, supported and helped where necessary. The tape required Jill to do two things:

1 Think of a pleasant subject on which to concentrate.
2 Tense and relax muscles in ascending sequence, from the feet to the head, under the guidance of the instructor until the whole body was relaxed, and she thought only of the pleasant subject.

She was told by the nurse to carry out the activity in a quiet, darkened area of the house where she was unlikely to be disturbed. It was also recommended that she lie down, either on the floor or her own bed.

The tape was played through and Jill obeyed the instructions, while Mother and the nurse observed. Afterwards they discussed her initial response to the tape and Jill explored her feelings concerning its effectiveness which she described as 'considerable'. At the end of the one hour visit Jill was set some homework. This consisted of a set of goals she had to achieve.

1 I will carry out the relaxation programme once each morning and once each afternoon.
2 I will monitor the length of time the relaxation remains after I have gone through the programme.
3 Should my peace of mind be interrupted, I will try to discover why and write it down.

During the next few weeks Jill was able to induce a state of relaxation in herself with quite a sustained after effect. Gradually the nurse showed her how to reduce her dependence upon the tape so that she carried out the technique using her own mental instructions. The nurse also began to introduce the subject of the least threatening item on Jill's list. Initially she simply brought it into the conversation to see how Jill would respond and, when the response was minimal, she brought it into open debate. It appeared that Jill had little or no anxiety to the idea of being at home on her own, but it might be quite different if she actually were on her own.

Desensitisation Programme

After the nurse had evaluated Jill's relaxation ability, it was felt that the time had come to begin tackling the items on the list, starting, as the nurse had already done, with the lowest. She explained that she intended to subject Jill, under controlled situations, to each item on the list. Jill was to practise her relaxation technique so that when confronted with the anxiety provoking situation she should be able to control her body's physical responses. She would be allowed to explore her feelings, with the nurse and Mother being supportive but firm with her. She would not be allowed to avoid a situation as this would only reinforce her fear. Also she would be expected to discuss the situation whilst subjected to it. Once she felt comfortable with one item, they would move on to the next one up the hierarchy. Each item represented a goal that she had to achieve and the behaviour necessary for her to do this would be repeated until she was no longer experiencing anxiety in that situation. Each goal was her personal contract, both with the

nurse and her mother and as with the relaxation homework, would be carried out regularly
in the absence of the nurse.

Each item was graded on three levels so that
in total there would be 30 goals to achieve
before Jill was able to go out on her own and
feel reasonably relaxed and comfortable. In
most cases it would also be necessary for the
third level goal to be carried out under supervision, or with help and support, before being
carried out on her own. This added a further
ten possible sub-goals to the list, making a
grand total of 40.

Sub-goals for each item on the hierarchy (arrows indicate height of anxiety)

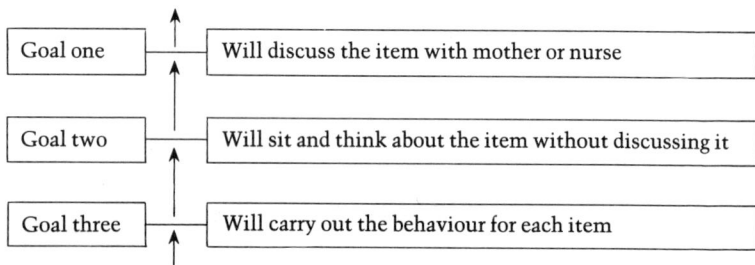

Goal one	Will discuss the item with mother or nurse
Goal two	Will sit and think about the item without discussing it
Goal three	Will carry out the behaviour for each item

Jill was told she must try to achieve the goals
for the first four items on the list, one per
week. This meant she was achieving a different sub-goal virtually every day. She was
alarmed at this but the nurse pointed out that
many of the first items were similar and she
needed to overcome them quickly so that she
could begin to enlarge upon her life activities.
It was also felt that the longer the process of
recovery took, the more difficult it would become. The first sub-goal was tackled at that
visit and Jill described her feelings, leaving the
nurse in little doubt that she was comfortable
and relaxed.

Subsequent sub-goals would be supervised
by Mother who seemed pleased to be a part of

the programme and was responding well to the challenge.

Evaluation

Each sub-goal and goal was evaluated by Jill herself, usually under guidance. She was asked to check the intensity of her responses by monitoring her physical feelings in response to the phobic items. The nurse evaluated Jill's progress by comparing her responses to those of the baseline observations she made at the beginning of the programme. Medication was regularly reviewed with Jill being asked when she felt she would like it to be reduced.

Finally no medication was used at all and the desensitisation programme progressed using Jill's learned control mechanisms as the only method of relaxation. The nurse might decide at a later date to bring Jill to the health centre for a weekly session rather than in the house so as to increase her desensitisation. At these meetings held by the nurse at the health centre she would discuss the feelings, problems, difficulties and successes she was experiencing with fellow sufferers. In this way she might hope to gain some insight into why she had responded in the way she had. The nurse would keep visiting at home for as long as the programme continued.

If progress became slow or non-existent, then alternative sub-goals would need to be devised which did not require so much from Jill. Also the items on the list might need to be changed as she became more aware of the exact nature of her fears.

1 What appears to be the relationship between a person's response to anxiety and his ability to function properly?
2 Why in the case study was it necessary for

the nurse to teach the process of relaxation before desensitisation took place?

3 Identify alternative methods of approaching the problems of a patient who is not able to achieve either their goals or subgoals.

4 The Skills of Counselling (1)

When people ask psychiatric nurses what they do, the reply usually involves a statement about establishing relationships and giving emotional support to those who are afraid, depressed, confused or disturbed. However, such a reply tells us little about exactly *how* the psychiatric nurse achieves these intentions. What do you do to build a relationship which leads to positive help and just how do you provide emotional support? If psychiatric nursing is really about these things, then we should be able to say what they are and how we achieve them.

The relationship between a person who needs help and the person willing to provide it is an area of such importance to the psychiatric nurse that it could be said to be at the very heart of nursing practice. Recognising the needs of some people who are in distress must be a central skill of the psychiatric nurse. Whilst the distressed person is in hospital, the contact he has with members of the caring team could be said to be fragmented as different nurses, occupational therapists, psychologists and doctors are all involved in the helping process at various times. Although they should all be following the same plan of intervention in his distress, it is inevitable that his degree and depth of relationship will vary from person to person. This can to some extent be at least partially overcome from a nursing relationship point of view by the primary nurse system which allows one nurse to be

Relationship in a nursing sense refers to interaction between people with the intention that helpful contact is developed over a period of time.

Primary nurse is a nurse who takes specific responsibility for nursing intervention from the beginning of one particular patient–nurse contact. This nurse should admit, interview, assess and plan the nursing for the patient and should be the patient's communication link with the caring team through to discharge and, in some cases, beyond.

at the centre of his care whilst others are peripheral to it.

In the community it is more common for one nurse (the CPN) to develop the special relationship which can be the key to providing real emotional support. The CPN is often the only nurse with whom the distressed person has frequent contact and, therefore, the relationship between them is of even greater importance. Indeed many CPNs look to one another for support in order to relieve the tension caused by this isolation.

The skills of building relationships and providing emotional support are central to the primary activity of counselling. It is in counselling we see the practice of nursing as psychiatric nurses themselves describe it when asked just what they do. So what is counselling?

A counselling model

Stage one — *The creation of an atmosphere characterised by:*
- Empathy
- Warmth
- Genuineness

Stage two — *Developing the relationship by:*
- Listening skills

Stage three — *Moving the relationship forward by:*
- Responding skills

One way of describing it can be as the process by which one person helps another by practising the skills of listening and responding within a relationship characterised by understanding, respect and human warmth.

Stage 1. In this first phase of establishing the counselling relationship it is vital to develop an atmosphere of empathy, warmth and genuineness.

Empathy means trying to see things through the other person's eyes rather than through our own, to try to understand how *he* feels rather than how *we* feel about him and his problems.

It's rather like trying to *be* the other person. If we continue to look at other people's problems from our own point of view, we are likely to see problems of our own rather than the ones which are distressing the person we want to help.

Seeing things from the nurse's point of view may lead to the development of sympathy for the other person; whilst this is not a bad thing, it is not as potent in helping as the development of empathy. Once the distressed person senses that the nurse is trying to understand him rather than feeling sorry for him, the relationship becomes fertile ground on which to sow the seeds of skilled help. This is achieved by the nurse keeping the emphasis and focus on the troubled person rather than on herself, and trying to understand how the other person feels by responding in such a way as to show this understanding. In the following example the nurse shows empathy by focussing on the patient's feelings and relays this to him in what she says:

Patient   'It's all so black, there's no way out of my problems.'
Nurse   'You feel trapped and despairing?'

Explanatory note: obviously it is important here that the nurse uses the right tone of voice in order to emphasise that she is trying to understand how he feels. Empathy, therefore, can be established by the nurse trying to see the meaning of what the patient says and feeding this back to him in such a way as to show understanding of his feelings rather than her own.

Warmth. If you have ever waited ages at a counter in a shop whilst the assistants carry on a conversation about their social lives rather than serve you, and eventually your money is taken from you and your purchase is thrown into a bag and thrust at you without a 'thank you', you will have some awareness of the importance of warmth in even the most superficial human interactions. Cold, detached shop assistants do not encourage return visits from their customers and most people would pay more money to be greeted with a smile and a friendly attitude.

The relationship between the CPN and the patient is one of considerably greater depth than the example given above and a lack of warmth can have more serious consequences than merely to make the patient look elsewhere for help. In a hospital the patient often has the opportunity to 'shop around' among the staff but in the community the options are reduced. In hospital, if the depressed person experiences difficulty in establishing a warm, friendly relationship with one nurse, he may find another, more rewarding nurse to associate with. When the patient is in his own home, the same community nurse visits regularly. He has little choice from a nursing point of view and may withdraw into himself if a satisfactory relationship cannot be established.

How then can the nurse show warmth to the distressed person? Firstly, being aware of the importance of non-verbal communication will enable the nurse to convey signs of friendliness and concern to the patient. The way the nurse sits with him, smiles, makes frequent eye contact and gives encouragement is vital to establishing a warm relationship. In other words the nurse must make a conscious, positive attempt to show warmth to the patient and the patient must feel this warmth coming from the nurse. Secondly, the nurse must concentrate on the patient and not on herself or on distractions in the environment.

Non-verbal communication is all communication between people which does not include the spoken word (but *does* include *tone* of voice).

Self awareness is the ability to recognise your own feelings and motives and their effects on other people.

Explanatory note: the issue of self awareness is important here and can help the nurse to give her full attention to the patient. For example, if the nurse hears something from the patient which triggers off a personal train of thought, she must be aware of this distraction and bring her thoughts back to the words the patient is saying and her attempts to read the feelings they express. By being aware of her own feelings, the nurse is better able to establish empathy and convey warmth to the person she wishes to help.

Genuineness. As warmth and empathy are vital in establishing a relationship between the nurse and any person requiring help, so the quality of genuine interest and concern for that person is also a key area. Genuineness involves developing respect for that person as an individual in his own right and unconditionally accepting the person for who he is. The CPN working in counselling is in a somewhat better position to establish this 'acceptance' because the distractions of the institutional environment and the dehumanising effects of such places are insignificant when the person is being helped on his own ground (at home).

The atmosphere for the creation of a relationship

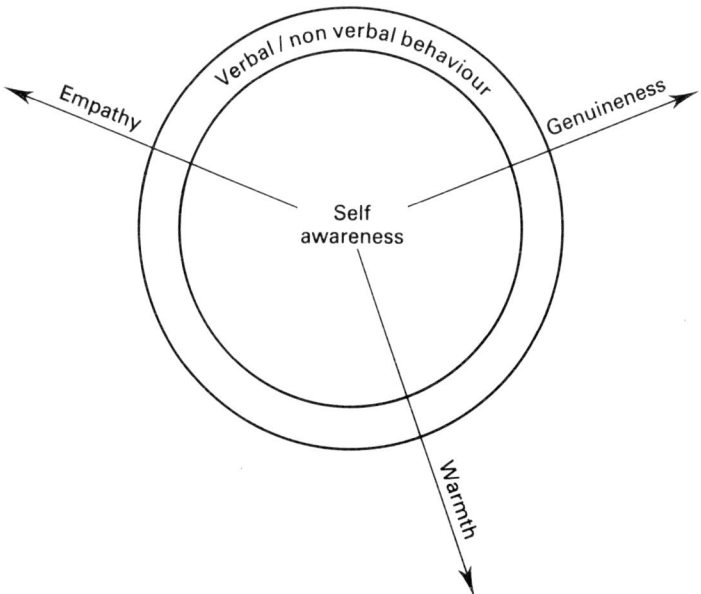

Obviously genuineness should not be faked; indeed the idea of such a thing is a contradiction in terms. Most people would soon see through a facade which tried to fool the troubled person into believing the concern was genuine and the relationship would be ruined. Pretending to be genuine is the province of the confidence trickster rather than the community psychiatric nurse. However, there are some techniques which allow the nurse to convey a feeling of genuine concern to the person; indeed if this is not relayed to the person, the relationship may never develop to a useful level.

The nurse can display genuineness by being consistent and dependable, and by giving time to the other person ungrudgingly. When an appointment is made for the community psychiatric nurse to call, the fact that she turns up on time and does not rush away at the first opportunity is evidence of her willingness to be with the patient. The practicalities of community psychiatric nursing often complicate this, and circumstances beyond the nurse's control will influence her ability to be dependable, but in the main the patient must be given time to feel secure in the relationship.

Genuineness is also felt within relationships by the development of trust in the other person. To some extent the traditional professional distance encouraged in nursing in the past has prevented the closeness that a real relationship demands. This can be overcome by the nurse being willing to 'risk' a deeper involvement in order to develop a genuine, empathic relationship with the patient. CPNs are rather more exposed (in the sense that they mostly work with the patient on a one to one basis) than the hospital nurse. It is vital that those nurses involved in developing such close relationships have the opportunity to meet regularly with each other in order to receive

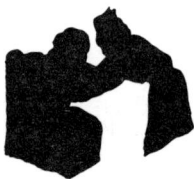

and give mutual advice and support.

In the second part of this chapter, we give an example of a CPN attempting to establish a warm, genuine, empathic relationship with a depressed person. The skills required for problem solving will be outlined and applied in the next chapter.

Arthur who Feels Depressed

HISTORY

For the last ten years Arthur had brought up his two children alone following the death of his wife in a car accident. Now, at 48, Arthur was experiencing a crisis in his life. Bringing up the two children had never been easy, especially as his job at the engineering factory had demanded much of his time and more so when he became charge-hand of his shift. Somehow he had managed to combine both parents' roles plus holding down a responsible job. He began to feel increasingly cut off from the outside world with little or no social contact beyond his work. As the children grew up, they needed him less and less and, despite quite a good relationship with his son Alan, Arthur was beginning to feel he no longer had anything to live for.

At work his job seemed relatively safe, yet these days that could never really be guaranteed. However, it was pretty obvious he was never going to get any more promotion. At home both his children spent less time with him, and his daughter, June, was becoming quite rebellious. Eventually, after several periods of sickness, Arthur had been seen by a psychiatrist at the request of his own GP. A period of hospitalisation had been recommended. At this time, Arthur was extremely depressed; he felt even more guilty at the thought of going into hospital and leaving his children to fend for themselves.

However, Arthur had progressed well in hospital and had recovered enough self-esteem and sense of purpose to return home to his children after only six weeks. Prior to leaving hospital, he had been visited on several occasions by the community psychiatric nurse, Derek Graham, who would be helping to support and guide him once discharged. They had developed quite a good relationship, both being keen football supporters and finding quite a lot to talk about outside their clinical roles.

Derek had taken Arthur home and helped him settle in, staying with him for a couple of hours whilst he orientated himself once again. Over the next few weeks, Derek visited once a week and felt quite confident of Arthur's recovery. He decided to extend the time between visits to two weeks, congratulating Arthur on his progress. They discussed ways in which he could extend his social life and gain further outlets for contact with others so it did not come as a surprise to find that he was out when Derek made the first fortnightly visit. Similarly, two weeks later when Arthur again was not at home, Derek was satisfied with his apparent improvement in social commitments. He spoke with the son, Alan, who said that his father often went out early in the evenings these days and seemed reasonably bright and cheerful. He did not say too much about how life was at home, and Derek did not push the matter.

However, on the third fortnightly visit, Derek was greeted at the door by a very concerned looking Alan who ushered him briskly into the house. He said that his father was upstairs and had been in bed for several days, refusing to come down. It had come to light that Arthur had not been out socialising at all but had been at his wife's grave, for several hours at a time. He had not attended work for over a week.

When Derek went upstairs, he found Arthur lying curled up in his bed. He sat with him for about ten minutes, trying to talk to him to find out what had happened, but Arthur refused to speak. Derek sat quietly by the bed for a few minutes telling Arthur that it was all right if he did not wish to speak to him, but that he was available if he should change his mind. He decided to question the son once again to see what had brought about this dramatic change in presentation. Telling Arthur that he would be downstairs if he wanted him, and that he

Initial approach to setting up Stage 1 of the counselling model

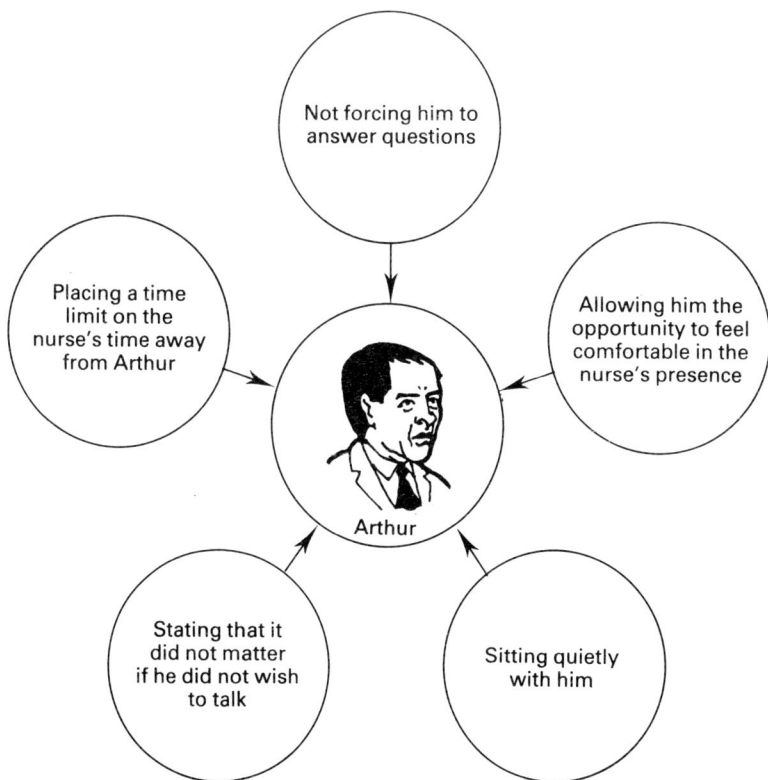

43

would only be five minutes, he went to see Alan.

Explanatory note: having ascertained that Arthur did not at that time wish to speak to him, it was essential that Derek did not simply walk away and leave him. This would have communicated lack of concern, frustration, boredom or simply the fact that he did not want to come to see Arthur, who was already feeling obvious anguish. To be rejected by Derek might only confirm for him what he already considered to be the case, namely that he was of no value to anyone, including himself. Despite wanting to talk to the son, Derek told Arthur that he would sit with him and that he was there should he need him. By doing so he communicated that he cared enough about Arthur to stay with him and that his caring was unconditional, in other words he expected nothing in return for sitting by his bed. After staying for a while he then told Arthur he was going downstairs, and could be contacted if necessary and stated an exact limit on his time away from the bed. In this way, he hoped to be able to show Arthur that he was still available and could be trusted to keep his word as he would make sure that he returned within the time limit. By doing this Derek, despite being unable to set up reciprocal communication, was creating an environment whereby counselling could begin to get at Arthur's understanding of his current problem.

Reciprocal communication is a communication between two individuals where each responds to the other spontaneously or without prompting.

Recent Developments

NURSING CARE

It became apparent from what Alan told Derek that the last few weeks had been very traumatic for his father. His job was in jeopardy and he discovered that his daughter was seeing a young boy notorious for being a bully, a vandal and a suspected solvent abuser. To top it all, Alan himself had decided to move away from home in an attempt to find work for himself. This meant that Arthur's world was being reshaped for him completely against his wishes. His apparent lack of control over external circumstances was enough to convince him that he was no longer of any good to anyone and, in particular, himself. The resul-

Solvent abuser is a person who uses various techniques to inhale the vapour of solvents such as glue, petrol, hair spray, etc. to gain an altered sense of awareness.

tant sadness he felt was his way of shutting himself away from it all.

Creating the Atmosphere for Counselling

Derek returned to Arthur when the five minutes had elapsed making sure that he was aware of his return within the stated time, but without making it too obvious. He knew that it was important to start Arthur talking, no matter how trivial the subject matter. He could begin to build on these interactions and eventually Arthur might be in a position to vent his feelings and begin to look more objectively at his life situation. The biggest problem was how to begin to get him to speak. Derek sat reasonably close to the bed in a relaxed pose in a position where Arthur could see him quite easily. He said that Arthur seemed tired and looked unhappy, and waited for a response from Arthur. He waited for several minutes and then said he thought that Arthur must be very sad. Arthur nodded his head in agreement, but said nothing verbally. Three further empathic approaches were followed with similar non-verbal responses:

Derek 'You seem to be troubled by what is going on around you.'
Arthur Nods in agreement.
Derek 'You feel it necessary to hide away from everything.'
Arthur Nods in agreement.
Derek 'You look very lonely.'
Arthur Nods in agreement.

At this point Derek felt the necessity to open the interaction. This being his final visit of the day, he had some time to spare and he said to Arthur, 'I have about an hour before I must leave. I will sit here with you. If you want to talk to me you can, but don't worry if you would rather not.' Arthur said, 'Thank you.'

Gradually during the next hour Arthur began to speak to Derek. True, he said very little about the way he felt and what had brought it all about, but at least he was making some form of verbal contact. When the hour was up, Derek excused himself, said he would return at a set time the next day, gave Arthur a telephone number where he could be contacted that evening if necessary, and left. Before leaving the house he suggested to Alan that he spend the evening sitting with his father, which he agreed to do, and spent a little time discussing the approach he had used and how Alan could adopt the same sort of strategy.

Explanatory note: the counselling process has not as yet begun in earnest. Hopefully the following visit would generate enough conversation to get at the heart of the matter and bring about some positive suggestions from Arthur as to how he could cope with his problems more successfully. Derek had not thought of re-admission as an approach for Arthur because he felt that it would only add to the problems he was already experiencing. The son was prepared to act as a counsellor in a minor way; if indeed he followed Derek's advice, he may well have a very profound effect upon Arthur's presentation, especially as he might well be part of Arthur's problem. The climate of counselling, however, had been set by Derek using a calm, warm, genuine and empathic approach towards Arthur and his apparent desire to remain silent.

| TEST YOURSELF |

1 In the counselling model identified in the text, what are the three basic components of Stage one?
2 Why was it necessary for the CPN to set limits on time spent away from Arthur?
3 What type of approach was the CPN using when he was trying to get Arthur to speak to him?

4   Why was re-admission to hospital not seen
     as a viable alternative in Arthur's case?

FURTHER READING

FRENCH, P. 1983. *Social Skills for Nursing Practice.* Beckenham: Croom Helm.

MUNRO, E., MANTHEI, R. & SMALL, J. 1983. *Counselling – a skills approach.* New Zealand: Methuen.

NELSON-JONES, R. 1983. *Practical counselling skills.* Eastbourne: Holt, Rinehart & Winston.

5 The Skills of Counselling (2)

In the previous chapter we described a model for counselling and stressed the importance of developing a relationship with the person in need which is based on warmth, empathy and genuineness. We now need to look at the skills the helper should use within this therapeutic relationship, to demonstrate their application in enabling people to gain perspective on their problems, and to develop possible solutions. It is important to remember throughout this chapter that the helping skills can only be really effective in most cases if time has been spent developing the relationship in the way described in the previous chapter.

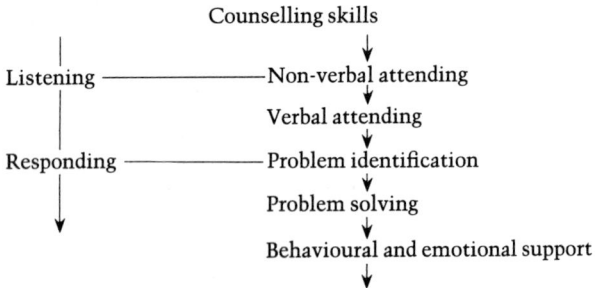

Counselling skills

Listening ———————————— Non-verbal attending

Verbal attending

Responding ———————————— Problem identification

Problem solving

Behavioural and emotional support

The skills of helping can generally be seen as falling into two major categories.

Listening Skills

Non-verbal attending. When we use the term non-verbal, we generally mean any method of communication between people which does not involve the spoken word, but which does include the tone of voice used. For example, laughing and crying can be described as non-verbal since they involve a high degree of body movement and facial expression, but no actual spoken words, even though noises are made.

How, then, can we show others that we are paying attention to them without actually speaking? This is important since trying to talk and listen at the same time is certainly unhelpful in the counselling situation. Indeed effective counsellors seem to do more listening than talking. Facing the other person squarely is a good method of helping them to realise you are concentrating on them. Sitting side by side only leads to sore necks for both parties.

It makes sense to want to see each other's face. The face is the main focus of attention in the counselling situation since it is through facial expression that we convey the emotions which back up our words. The eyes in particular provide potent signals, and frequent eye contact is very important in human communication. Whilst intense staring at the other person can be counterproductive and rather threatening, it is essential that face to face contact involve the positive expressions of smiling and nodding at regular and appropriate intervals. Frequent eye contact is better than continuous intense staring.

The posture adopted by the helper is also an important non-verbal method of letting the other person know he is being listened to. Sitting in an open relaxed posture is more encouraging than sitting with arms and legs crossed. Leaning toward the other person will emphasise the helper's wish to concentrate on what is being said.

Explanatory note: Non-verbal attending is a listening skill which involves sitting squarely and openly facing the other person, and making frequent, positive eye contact. The aim of this conscious activity is to encourage the other person to talk freely in the security of knowing he is with a person who *wants* to listen.

Verbal attending. If you are communicating with someone by telephone, the use of non-verbal methods is greatly reduced (you are generally restricted to such 'non-words' as 'oh', 'mm', and 'ah'). If no verbal response is forthcoming from the other end of the line, the conversation may soon dry up due to lack of confirmation that the other person is actually listening. So verbal attending can be seen as the practice of using words and phrases to encourage the other person to continue, to confirm for them that they are being noted. Verbal attending makes no attempt to solve people's problems; problem identification and coping comes at a later stage.

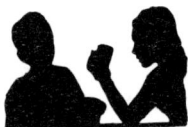

The nurse can let the other person know he is being listened to by frequently repeating the content of what is being said and rephrasing it into other words. This is known as reflecting and is a verbal skill used by most people without realising it. It is also useful to summarise the conversation, especially when it seems the patient is becoming a little confused about what he is saying. For example, after the patient has been talking for a while, the nurse might say: 'You've said that your drinking has caused you to feel very guilty and that most of your family seem to have lost sympathy for you.'

The patient can now confirm or deny this as an accurate summary of what he has been saying, and the conversation can move on in the knowledge that both parties see the situation in the same way.

Explanatory note: If the nurse asks questions in such a way as to show understanding of the conversation's content, the relationship begins to develop in a positive, progressive manner. In this way, verbal attending is evidence for the patient which confirms he is being listened to; if this were not the case, the nurse would be unable to reflect, summarise or question appropriately.

Responding Skills

Problem identification. Many people know they feel troubled but are unable to put their finger on just what things in their lives are making them feel that way. The nurse's role in this respect is to help the patient order his thoughts and recognise exactly what factors represent problems for him.

This can be facilitated by getting the patient to speak about things *he* sees as upsetting him, and by attaching priority to these factors, according to their power over him. Once this is done, he may be able to see more clearly and specifically which particular things represent real problems and, even more importantly, that they are *his* problems and therefore that the solutions to them must come from him.

Problem solving. Having identified which particular aspects of concern are of most importance to the patient, the nurse can then help him to look at ways of overcoming them. A useful way of doing this is to set a goal which represents a successful solution, and to then identify factors which will help achieve that goal. At the same time hindering influences can be identified and a plan to reduce them produced. In the example below, a person was asked about his strategies to reduce his drinking and a plan of action was drawn up based on positive and negative influences identified with the help of a nurse. In this method (sometimes referred to as Force Field Analysis), the influences listed under the helping column can be increased whilst those under the hindering column can be reduced. Obviously things are often not as simple as they first

A person who **facilitates** provides opportunities for the other person to help himself rather than being lead into making decisions he does not actually want to make.

appear, and no easy solutions to hindering influences may be identified. The advantage of this exercise is that both the nurse and the patient can look together at influences on which they both agree; this serves as a basis for behavioural change. It gives the nurse the opportunity to use skills in the therapeutic areas of anxiety management, self awareness, assertion training and relaxation techniques. These are all dealt with in other chapters in this book.

Goal setting in problem solving

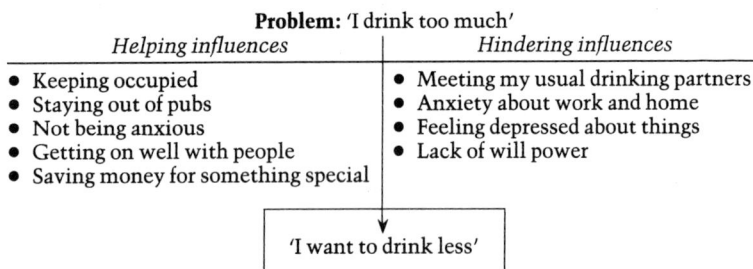

Problem: 'I drink too much'

Helping influences	*Hindering influences*
• Keeping occupied	• Meeting my usual drinking partners
• Staying out of pubs	• Anxiety about work and home
• Not being anxious	• Feeling depressed about things
• Getting on well with people	• Lack of will power
• Saving money for something special	

'I want to drink less'

Behavioural and Emotional Support

Positive reinforcement. Rewarding behaviour which achieves a positive result nearly always encourages repetition and continuation of that behaviour.
A contract is an agreement between nurse and patient that certain behaviour will occur between counselling sessions and that a specific goal will be achieved by a pre-agreed time.

The nurse's role in helping the patient achieve the goals he sets for himself centres around giving positive support to actions he takes which reduce hindering influences and increase helping ones. This can be achieved by the use of positive reinforcement, and by making a contract for improvement which forms the basis for future counselling sessions. During this period, it is important that the nurse represent a positive influence for the patient and that occasional lapses are understood and seen to be only setbacks, rather than total failures. The relationship between the nurse and patient is, to some extent, under the microscope at this stage and the work done to establish warmth, empathy and genuine concern is repaid by satisfaction for both parties.

HISTORY

Malcolm who has lost his control of alcohol

Malcolm Harris was 32 years old, married with two children and unemployed. On three separate occasions in the past, he had been admitted to the acute psychiatric ward of his local general hospital with problems which had made him depressed. On each of these admissions, he had always been drinking heavily and it was known that he had difficulty controlling the amount of alcohol he consumed. Indeed, he had lost at least one job through a series of events that were linked to alcohol abuse.

Alcohol abuse is drinking to excess (often leading to drunkenness) to avoid facing up to problems.

The CPN was visiting Malcolm as the necessary follow up on his progress since his last discharge. He had been out for nearly two months and appeared to be doing quite well. He was alert, quite active, looking for work and seemed to be getting on well with his wife. Unfortunately, he was still drinking, and at times quite heavily. He was not on any form of medication so there was no danger of the alcohol having any serious effects upon him from that angle, but when the home situation was studied closely, it was obvious that the drinking was dramatically affecting his ability to function satisfactorily as a husband and parent.

NURSING CARE

Active Listening

At first the nurse did not recognise the extent of the problem. It was only when the conversation lead to the day to day activities in which

53

Malcolm was involved that a potential problem area was identified. He stated that he was always doing odd jobs around the house to keep busy, but his wife said he was more likely to be found at the pub. Malcolm grinned uneasily at this and tried to pass it off as a joke, but his wife persisted and in a flood of words, told how he drank most of their money away, never did anything around the house and was rude and aggressive towards their two children. Malcolm denied all of this and his wife stormed out of room, crying.

Explanatory note: very often verbal and non-verbal clues as to the real significance of the information being collected are inconsistent with the actual information itself. In Malcolm's case the nurse simply allowed the conversation to wander where it would, picking out the important elements within it and stringing them together to form a pattern. On the one hand Malcolm stated he was well and coping; on the other his wife said he was not and gave reasons why. Which one was true, and what should be done about it? Obviously there was no necessity for the wife to make the story up, and as she had been supportive throughout Malcolm's difficult periods, it was fair to assume that what she said had an element of truth about it. Malcolm was adamant that he was not behaving the way his wife suggested and, indeed, she might be exaggerating. The nurse, therefore, needs to establish the exact nature of the problem.

Conflicting information for the nurse to unravel

Husband	*Wife*
• I do not have a drink problem	• You do have a drink problem
• I work around the house	• You do nothing around the house
• I have a good relationship with my family	• You behave badly towards our children
• I am telling the truth	• You are lying
• I do not need help	• I want something done
• I am OK	• I am upset by your behaviour

Nurse

Responding: Problem Identification

By simply being available at the time of a crisis, the nurse has established that a problem exists which might otherwise have remained hidden. However, he is now faced with two difficulties of his own:

1   He needs to help Malcolm admit to the existence of an alcohol related problem.
2   He needs to identify both the cause and the consequence of the problem if he is to help Malcolm and his family find a way of dealing with it successfully.

The nurse questioned Malcolm as to why his wife should make such statements. He had to do so in such a way as to seem neutral, neither believing nor disbelieving, so as not to antagonise him. He did this using an open-ended questioning technique. In this way, Malcolm was allowed the opportunity to freely discuss his own feelings, both about his wife's statement and his own behaviour. It became apparent that Malcolm felt the need to hide his true feelings concerning certain matters because he used obfuscation whenever they came into conversation. However, the nurse noted the areas of concern and decided a more direct approach was necessary at this point.

Open-ended questioning technique is asking questions which do not have any specific answer thus enabling the individual to talk about whatever he feels important or significant.
Obfuscation is a technique used in discussion which seeks to mislead the listener or confuse the issue.

Explanatory note: open-ended questioning is very useful for allowing the patient to determine the content of conversation. The listener can then identify those areas most disturbing for the patient. Unwittingly, if allowed, we all tend to wander unintentionally in conversation to those areas which have the most effect upon us. It is often a totally unconscious process. A skilled listener is usually quite able to detect those areas of concern even though they may not have been fully clarified by the speaker. It is almost as if we desperately need to talk about what is troubling us, yet cannot consciously bring ourselves to do so, for whatever reason, shame, embarrassment, guilt, etc. Yet our brain deceives us, and brings the subjects out into the open, even as we speak. This was the case with Malcolm. He is obviously troubled by his drinking and its effects upon his family, yet he cannot discuss it openly because it would be admitting some sort of failure. He therefore gives little clues to the nurse who collects them together and is able to focus directly onto them. The most important thing for the nurse to do at this point is to help the patient see them for himself rather than simply be told of their existence. This may take a long time and should not be hurried.

The nurse asked Malcolm how much alcohol he drank each day, when he drank it, if he drank more at certain times than at others, and what happened as a consequence of drinking it. From the answers it was clear he drank to become drunk, and usually when he and his wife had been arguing about marital and household problems. Malcolm admitted as much himself as a result of the direct questioning and spoke at great length about his fears, his worries and his own interpretation as to why he drank so much.

Direct questioning is asking specific questions which call for a specific answer. Often used to pin point exact problem areas and particularly useful in helping the speaker to concentrate his ideas and feelings.

It was necessary for the nurse to get Malcolm to consider the real reasons for abusing alcohol. He asked him to write down the occasions in the past few weeks when he had become drunk, and what had happened between him and his wife before doing so. He said that he would call the next day and discuss the list with Malcolm. Lastly he asked him not to have any alcohol between now and their next meeting. Malcolm agreed. Thus Malcolm had to take some responsibility for his own behaviour, making a contract with the nurse which only he could keep.

NURSING CARE

Problem Tackling

When the nurse visited the next day, Malcolm had kept to his contract, having not had any alcohol, and produced his list of dates for discussion. The nurse asked him to consider them and analyse what they meant. Malcolm readily admitted that he only seemed to get drunk when his wife made him feel unimportant and lazy, or threatened his self esteem.

Force field analysis of Malcolm's problem

Malcolm
Problem: 'I drink when I feel threatened'

Helping influences	*Hindering influences*
• Talking to my wife about the way I feel • Staying in the house • Doing jobs around the house • Playing with the children • Actually looking for employment • Helping my wife get things done • Being praised by my wife	• Not talking to anyone • Going to the pub • Being inactive • Watching the TV • Getting jealous of other people who seem to be happy • Feeling frustrated about my life • Shutting my children out of my life • Feeling guilty about not having a job

'I will not drink when I argue with my wife'

It was agreed that both he and the nurse should construct a list of factors which help and hinder his desire to overcome the need for alcohol.

NURSING
CARE

Behavioural and Emotional Support

The two of them discussed the negative influences, how they could be avoided, how they could be overcome and why they seemed to have such a disruptive effect. They also discussed how the positive influences could be used to offset those which heightened his desire to drink. His wife was asked to join in with the discussion so that she did not become ostracised by the proceedings. It was important that both she and Malcolm felt that they had responsibility in helping Malcolm achieve his goal because they would be able to support each other, provide guidance and positive reinforcement on a mutual basis. By sharing the recovery programme, much of the burden of guilt which both of them might feel could be effectively dealt with.

They decided to look at their own relationship, their worries and fears, highlights and problems, and consider them in the light of Malcolm's drinking. In this way they hoped to identify factors which sparked off the desire for alcohol. The nurse had to establish a contract with Malcolm that would sustain him until his next visit. It would also act as a mini goal; if it is achieved the nurse can reward Malcolm with warmth and encouragement. It was agreed that he would only drink alcohol in small amounts when in the company of his wife, and only if they had not been arguing.

Follow up Visits

NURSING CARE

Over the next few months, the nurse visited Malcolm on numerous occasions. They agreed many contracts, not all of which were kept, but the nurse never criticised Malcolm. Gradually, as he grew to like himself a little more and gained something positive from his life, Malcolm's difficulty with alcohol became less of a problem. As the desire for alcohol diminished, seeking worthwhile employment became more of a challenge. The nurse had to ensure that each component in Malcolm's life which appeared to generate feelings of helplessness and frustration were examined and dealt with using the Force Field approach, so reducing the chance that disappointment would lead to a repetition of his drinking problems.

TEST
YOURSELF

1 What are the main components in the counselling programme that enable problems to be identified and tackled by the person who suffers them?
2 How does Force Field analysis benefit both the patient and the nurse when considering problem solving?
3 Explain why the nurse needs to reinforce positive behaviour exhibited by the patient.

FURTHER
READING

EGAN, G. 1975. *The Skilled Helper.* Wadsworth: Belmont, Ca.
PRIESTLY, P., MCQUIRE, J., FLEGG, D., HEMSLEY, V. & WELHAM, D. 1978. *Social Skills and Personal Problem Solving.* London: Tavistock.

6 The Skills of Reality Orientation

If there is one specific area of psychiatric care where criticism of the institutional approach has been loud and consistent, it is in the care of the elderly mentally ill. Caring for this group of people has often been seen as unrewarding by newly qualified staff who prefer to become involved in work considered more dynamic and progressive. The occupants of the psycho-geriatric ward do not represent the idea of psychiatric nursing with which most potential students and pupils arrive at the initial interview for the job, and first placement on the geriatric wards comes as a rude awakening to many. Whilst some nurses find that involvement with the elderly proves to be the type of work they enjoy, the majority move on to more popular areas of psychiatry, leaving the wards staffed by only a few trained nurses and with the shortfall made up by nursing auxiliaries. Good though many auxiliaries are, surely the care of the elderly mentally ill is important enough to warrant the commitment of trained nursing staff?

Confusion is a state which can occur in clear consciousness, and is characterised by muddled thinking shown outwardly in behaviour and speech content. It is commonly seen in elderly people and is often the result of treatable physical disorder.

The important point to emphasise is how vital it is to avoid carrying such a negative point of view into the community, where many old, confused people are cared for by loving friends and relatives and our profession is looked to as a positive support resource.

Explanatory note: the role of the CPN in the care of the elderly is to participate in a joint approach which involves both professional and voluntary contributions. In good hospital wards and old peoples' homes, this co-operation already exists, but unfortunately it does not

Disorientation is
being unaware of
the correct time,
place and/or
person.

appear to be the norm. It is still quite easy to find rooms full of dishevelled, disorientated and incontinent elderly people for whom the evening of life is miserable and pointless.

So how can the CPN bring professional skills and positive attitudes to this important area of care?

Firstly, the skills needed are those of providing a high standard of sensitive assistance to the relative who has decided to care for the elderly person at home. Close co-operation and consultation must be the corner stone of this important relationship.

Secondly, the attitude of the CPN to the elderly person must be of a positive nature. This is characterised by respect for that person as an individual with needs which are just as important as those of a younger person.

One particular area of skilled help for the elderly, confused and disorientated is an approach known as Reality Orientation. As the name implies, the emphasis in this psychological approach is on helping the person to stay in touch with the world around them by aiding orientation in time, space and person. It tries to prevent the downward spiral so often seen in psychological functioning among the elderly mentally infirm by encouraging awareness of the reality of the environment.

Explanatory note: as a psychological technique, *reality orientation* originated in the United States during the 1950s, but since it is true that there is 'nothing new under the sun', it would be safe to assume that many people had practised it on this side of the Atlantic without giving it quite as much thought as its refined use now merits.

What is Reality Orientation?

The basic essentials of reality orientation are the systematic, consistent relaying of current

Reinforcement is following up an action with a reward or a punishment. The action can then be seen as positive or negative. Positively reinforced behaviour is likely to be repeated by the recipient.

Attitude is a tendency to respond to an object, situation, or idea in some preferential manner. Attitudes are based on the values we hold about things.

information about the environment, such as time, weather conditions, identity and surroundings, whilst not reinforcing any sign of irrational or confused thinking. This means more than having a large blackboard in the corner of the room with the date written on it. Although such provision is well intended, it hardly represents reality, since few of us would like to have such an object in our living room. A large calendar with a picture appropriate to the season displayed prominently can be the object of carefully directed attention by the person helping to maintain orientation. The important point is the emphasis of reality rather than the construction of an artificial environment which might resemble it.

Holden and Woods (1982) identify three major components of reality orientation:

1 Basic, informal reality orientation
2 Intensive reality orientation
3 Attitude therapy

In the first approach, the important factor is a consistent continual input from the helper to allow orientation to the environment to be maintained by directing the person to clues around them. The second approach requires a more structured, planned set of sessions directed toward reinforcing the basic, informal work and extending it into areas not covered so intensively during the former. Attitude therapy is chiefly concerned with the identification of specific attitudes on the part of the elderly person and the helper in order to achieve an appropriate consistent approach.

Reality orientation has largely been used with in-patients but its application to a community setting is possible and very useful. Either by forming small groups at day centres or by helping relatives to develop skills for use with the elderly person at home, the CPN can make a positive and important contribution to applying the technique outside the hospital environment. By virtue of the CPN's knowledge and skills in teaching, the relative can be taught to use basic reality orientation between the intensive sessions conducted by the nurse and/or other therapists. For example, the CPN can arrange for intensive groups to be held at a health centre, and can help train the caring relative in the skills to be used between attendances. By doing this, shared responsibility becomes the cornerstone of care and the relationship between the patient–relative–nurse becomes a positive factor in the overall approach. For a deeper, yet clearly stated account of the underlying principles of this cooperation, the reader is referred to the excellent work of Holden and Woods (1982).

HISTORY

Emily who has become confused in late life

Emily is 74 years old and lives with her eldest daughter and her family. She has two other children, both sons, and for the past few years since the death of her husband, she has lived for one yearly periods in the homes of each of these three children. In this way she has enjoyed a varied and caring home situation in the community where she has spent the vast majority of her life. Her children have had the satisfaction of seeing her grow old gracefully amongst those she knows and loves yet, by sharing the problems of accommodation among themselves, have been able to reduce the added stress that an elderly parent can so often bring to a family.

Recently Emily has become increasingly muddled in her thoughts and forgetful about all manner of personal things. In fact her recent memory has become quite impaired and has led to her being unable to contribute to the

Recent memory is the ability of an individual to recall events that have taken place anything from a few moments ago, to those of last year.

social interactions within the home in the way she has done over the years. Increasingly she forgets people's names, dates, places and then incorrectly identifies the room she is in, who people are on the television, times, relatives and events, etc. Her daughter and son-in-law have found it difficult to come to terms with this change in her presentation because it has added to the amount of 'looking after' that she requires. Everything has to be explained in far greater detail, often having to be repeated several times before it appears to be understood by Emily. As a result of this, everyone has become a little irritable and agitated with the result that Emily has begun to withdraw from her role as family member to one of outside observer.

The daughter contacted her GP who made a domiciliary visit to assess Emily in the confines of her home environment. He referred the situation to the CPN because he felt that despite the absence of any previous psychiatric history, Emily was showing considerable deterioration in her general mental functioning.

General mental functioning is the individual's ability to perform single mental activities such as remembering, analysing, orientating and logical thinking in a spontaneous fashion.

Explanatory note: it is more usual for an elderly person to exhibit behaviour consistent with abnormal ageing at an earlier age than in Emily's case. However, it is often the case that the deterioration of general mental functioning is not so obviously apparent when the individual is nursed or cared for by their own relatives and in their own homes. This is because of the constant companionship they receive, the love and warmth consistent with family life, and the general tolerance exhibited by one's own family. Had Emily been in an institutional set up, it is quite possible that signs of deterioration would have been detected much earlier and the degree of decline been far more rapid.

First Visit

The CPN who visited Emily specialised in the care of the elderly in the community and was therefore skilled in the assessment techniques necessary to establish the level of Emily's mental decline. She measured Emily's ability to remember and recall simple events, such as the day, the date, the time and place. She asked about well known people such as the Prime Minister, the Queen, and other

The CPN's evaluation of Emily's behaviour at the first visit

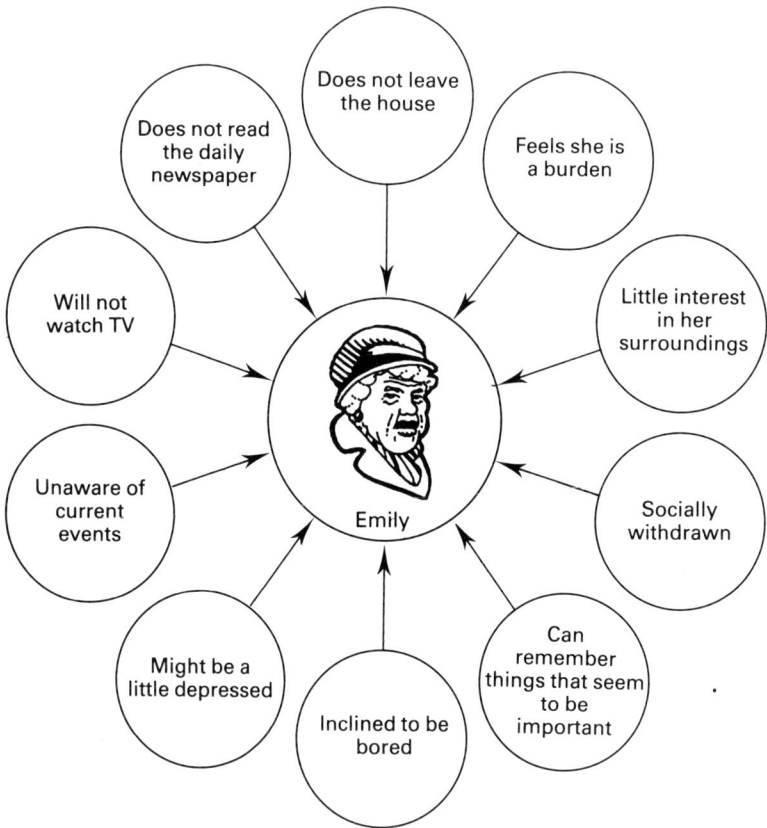

Does not read the daily newspaper

Does not leave the house

Feels she is a burden

Will not watch TV

Little interest in her surroundings

Unaware of current events

Emily

Socially withdrawn

Might be a little depressed

Inclined to be bored

Can remember things that seem to be important

65

members of the Royal Family. She asked Emily to hold her bag for her whilst she went out of the room and on return wanted to see if Emily could remember that it belonged to the nurse. She noted her reluctance to indulge in conversation, and her general lack of awareness of current events. However, she concluded that Emily appeared to be measurably well orientated but seemed to be suffering more from the effects of boredom or sensory deprivation rather than chronic brain failure (*senile dementia*). She discussed her findings with the daughter, and it was generally agreed that a programme of re-integration should be pursued including, in particular, the process of reality orientation.

Nurse's Role

NURSING CARE

It was obvious that Emily's family were prepared to help with the provision of care and support but their difficulty lay in not knowing what to do for the best. The nurse had already established that Emily was becoming withdrawn because she found the world either uninteresting or even a little frightening. It was important, therefore, that she regain her interest and confidence in a way that was both stimulating and therapeutic. To do this it would be necessary to re-introduce her to the world around her in such a way as to generate real and natural feelings of interest that did not seem to emanate simply from a contrived, clinical situation. The process of reality orientation could be carried out effectively by the nurse, but only on a very restricted basis because of the time available to actually spend with Emily. Also, because Emily was not exhibiting a picture of an individual rapidly on the decline, it was safe to conclude that she would not need much professional input for the present if her relatives were taught properly how to cope with her immediate needs. The nurse would, therefore, discuss with them how to go about bringing Emily back into contact with the real world that existed all around her and out of the one she was beginning to construct for herself within her own mind.

Explanatory note: at a later date in the proceedings, when Emily had begun to regain some of her confidence, it might be deemed a good idea if she attended regular sessions of reality orientation within a group setting at the health centre. In this way, she would meet others of her own age, in the same situation as herself and with similar backgrounds. She would be able to expand her social connections as well as allowing the nurse to monitor her progress in a relatively controlled environment. It would be wrong to start Emily's programme in such a way because as yet she was still unsure of herself and her surroundings (hence the development of some of her behaviour). Once she had begun to regain some of her personal skills and the zest for involvement once again, it might be necessary for the nurse to discuss with the three children their accommodation roster. It was obvious that although the living with each of her children for yearly periods on a rotational basis had been fine for several years, it was not what Emily wanted now. The problem was that she might not know it herself, nor might she be prepared to approach her children about her fear of rejection or even retribution.

The nurse discussed the setting up of orientation facilities within the home, explaining that the rationale for such activities was the need to bring Emily back into the world as it is right now. It was therefore necessary to ensure that in Emily's room she had a calendar with a large geographic photograph depicting the current climate. In this way, Emily should be able to identify the approximate time of the year before she considered what day it actually was. The need for accurate visual representations is important, pictures, drawings, photographs, etc., especially if they are striking

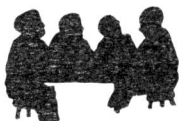

and bold. They would catch Emily's eye in a way that mere words could never do. As the nurse explained to the daughter, words to Emily tend to merge into the background, thus becoming as passive as that background. They are only a method of code after all, and have to be converted by the brain into a visual picture of what they denote. If you cut out the words and go straight to the picture, half the problem of identification is already complete.

Elements of Emily's home orientation programme

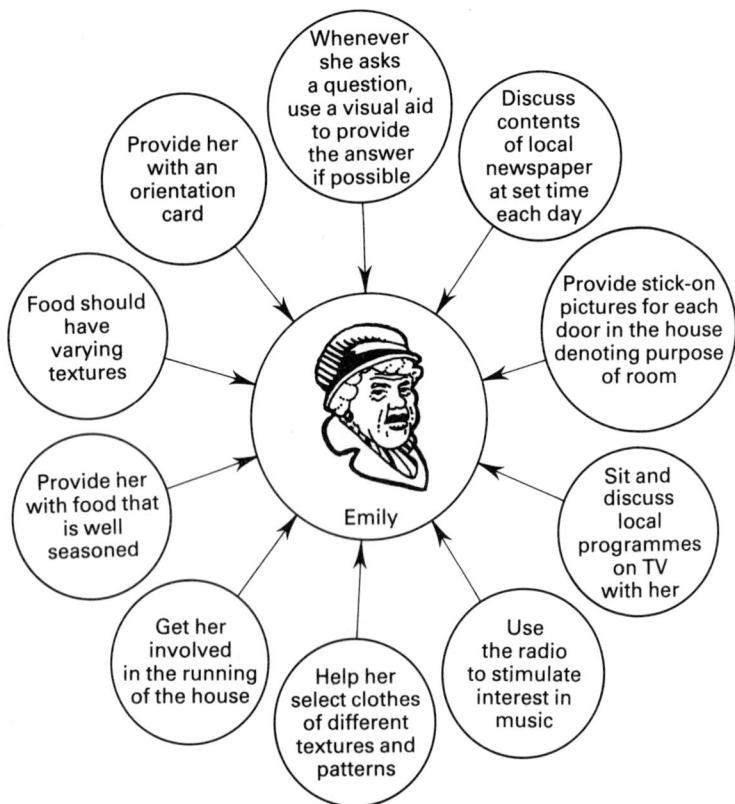

General Approach

The need to provide a stimulating and varied environment in which to live was stressed, and Emily's daughter was told how to help her mother make use of the facilities around her. She was shown how necessary it was not to simply answer questions put to her by Emily, but to reinforce the answer in some way, either by directing her attention to something which illustrated what she was saying, or by developing a discussion in which Emily was guided into answering the question for herself. It is important that Emily does as much for herself as possible without it seeming as if others were rejecting her. The daughter would need considerable patience at first, but as Emily developed more of an awareness of her surroundings once again, the pressure would begin to ease.

It was also suggested that, amongst all the other orientation activities, her daughter should give Emily an orientation card at the beginning of each day. She could either put it beside her mother's bed each morning and ensure that she had it with her throughout the day, or actually give it to her, pointing out what it said upon it. At regular intervals during the day, she could ask her mother about the contents of the card, what it said, etc. so that she was constantly reminded of the data it contained. She must, of course, ensure that it was updated each day.

The nurse also invited the daughter to visit a weekly session of the reality orientation group at the health centre so that she would have some idea of how the process was carried out. In this way, she could hear useful ideas from the nurse who acted as therapist for the group.

An orientation card is a small card that can be placed either in a handbag, a pocket or wallet, that has basic details about the day, special appointments, things to do, what year it is, your address, etc.

Evaluation of Emily's progress

Emily's progress would be evaluated both on a formal and an informal basis. Her daughter was asked to monitor the overall effects of the programme on the way her mother behaved in the home. She was also asked to assess her mother's ability to answer straightforward questions about general awareness, such as the year, the name of the Prime Minister, the month, etc. In turn, the nurse would visit Emily once a fortnight initially for about a half an hour to simply sit and talk with her. During these visits, she would formally re-evaluate Emily's performance against that of the baseline observation she made at the initial visit. As she explained to the daughter, she could not be absolutely sure that her mother was going to improve because of this form of intervention, but she could be reasonably sure that the deterioration could be slowed down. Only the orientation programme itself would be able to supply the answer. However, it was important that the daughter be as creative as possible whenever it came to providing new ideas. If her mother did not seem to be responding to a particular approach, she must not automatically conclude that she was getting worse; it could be, after all, that the daughter had not selected a particularly good method of dealing with the problem. Lastly she was told that, should she have any difficulties with the programme or need advice or assistance in dealing with a particular problem, she could contact the nurse at the health centre directly.

The programme was designed to help Emily regain her personal confidence and improve the quality of her life. To do this, she had to develop some of her independence once again, so the nurse would only involve herself on the periphery for the immediate future, and would not interfere with the daughter's home life, unless asked to do so by the daughter herself. The programme, of course, was also designed to help Emily's family cope with the problem of caring for an elderly, tired and seemingly bored parent, who in other situations may well have been unnecessarily admitted to a ward for the elderly mentally ill.

TEST YOURSELF

1 What are the three basic approaches to reality orientation?
2 Why is it particularly necessary for an elderly individual to orientate themselves correctly?
3 How might relatives, friends and possibly voluntary organisations be involved in the setting up of an orientation programme for an individual in their own home?
4 What are the basic requirements for an effective home orientation programme?

FURTHER READING

HOLDEN, U. & WOODS, R. 1982. *Reality Orientation: Psychological approaches to the confused elderly.* Edinburgh: Churchill Livingstone.
RIMMER, J. 1982. *Reality Orientation, principles and practice.* Buckinghamshire: Winslow Press.

7 The Skills of Crisis Intervention

Crisis is a period of emotional upset related to a specific situation which has threatened the stability of the person. It involves the feeling that the means to cope are not present and can lead to helplessness and emotional breakdown.

When a person in hospital experiences a personal crisis or if a personal crisis has lead to hospital admission, there are many resources on hand to aid in coping. Doctors, nurses, psychologists, voluntary workers and many others are almost immediately available to provide professional support. In the community, the available help is less easily summoned and many people, whether ex-patients or those who have never been in hospital, can feel isolated and helpless. It is therefore important that a community psychiatric nurse should be skilled in recognising the emerging crisis situation and be able to give help and summon assistance on behalf of the troubled person.

We all have the basic mechanism to cope with physical threat and we do not have to learn to bring this machinery into use. If you are walking along the path and a person jumps out of a doorway and attacks you, it is very difficult to avoid bringing into play some physical reaction, whether it means fighting back or running away. However, we do tend to base our reaction on previous experiences which have been successful, and a confident judo expert is more likely to fight than run away. Psychological threats, such as that posed by the sudden loss of someone held dear to you, can often evoke a similar response to a physical threat and reactions are dictated by how you have coped with similar situations in the past. If you have been successful in coping with emotional upset, you are likely to bring those successful tactics into play again, but if past experience has been unpleasant or has lacked success, you may feel ill-equipped to deal with the problem. Crisis reaction can follow.

What is a Crisis Reaction?

Mostly it seems to be a state of anxiety, helplessness and despondency, but many special-

The phases of a crisis

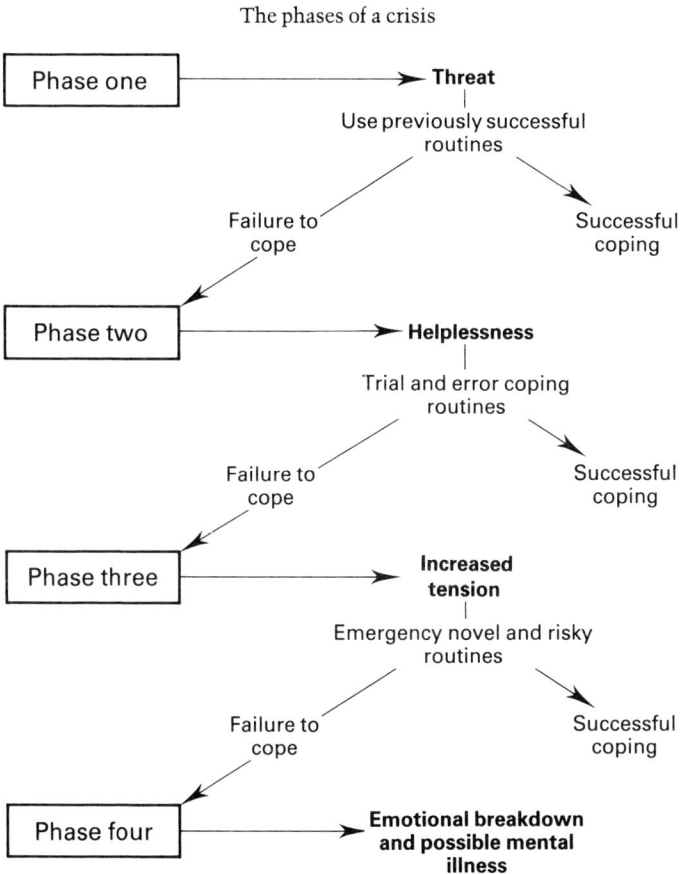

ists have identified specific stages in this reaction and it is by recognising them that the CPN can play a big part in helping people to cope. Murgatroyd and Woolfe (1982) outline one sequence of stages based on the work of G. Caplan. It can be seen that the person seems to respond to an emotional threat, such as personal loss, by either coping or failing to cope at critical points; continual failure can result in a downward emotional collapse and the possible development of a mental illness. How can the CPN intervene in crisis situations? There seem to be two major areas.

Intervention is 'stepping in' as a positive action designed to use the person's own resources as a means to coping with the problem.

Firstly, the CPN can help emotionally and materially when it has been forecast that a crisis may occur. For example, a person who has been subject to bouts of severe anxiety and depression whenever separated from her mother may well need pre-crisis intervention if hospital investigations indicate that her mother may die. The CPN in this case will need to prepare her for the expected crisis that bereavement may provoke. This help can be given in the form of discussion linked to the delivery of psychological support and a realistic approach to the potential problem. The relationship the CPN has established with the person in the past can have a profound influence on the effectiveness of help offered at this stage.

Secondly, the community psychiatric nurse can intervene once the crisis has actually occurred and the person is involved in the process described earlier. The activities here are similar, in that support and encouragement to face the problem and open discussion of the person's feelings are essential ingredients, but an extra dimension is present as the troubled person is likely to be even more dependent and the feeling of inability to cope is probably stronger. The objective in this stage of crisis intervention must be to help the person keep a realistic perspective of what the problems are *now* rather than a negative view of past inabilities to cope with similar problems.

Before we give an example of a CPN intervening in a personal, emotional crisis which occurred within a family as a result of one member becoming psychiatrically disturbed at home, it may be useful to summarise the basic principles involved:

1 A crisis can be a positive experience if the skills used to resolve it are learnt and can be applied to a similar situation should it arise. However, frequent experience of failure to cope can lead to recurring crises and a long-term dependency. Therefore it is essential that the CPN should help the person successfully resolve the problem in order to prevent future situations producing more and more dependency.

2 A crisis is usually related to life experiences which are generally seen as significant by the person and, therefore, their occurrence may be predictable.

Significant life events are any specific event which has significance for the person, e.g. bereavement, failing an important examination or being made redundant.

3 Any help must concentrate on what is happening now and how the person feels *now*. There is no profit for the person or the helper indulging in deep analysis of what may be underlying the problem. There is more time for that sort of analytic behaviour once the crisis is over.

4 The nurse must help the person face the realities of the situation and not aid and abet attempts to escape by running away from the problem, however tempting that action may be. As was said in point 1, positive learning can only take place if the crisis is coped with rather than avoided.

5 The CPN is part of a team and should make full use of others within that team who may be able to help when the situation demands it. It

is not an admission of failure if assistance is requested when necessary.

6 Counselling skills outlined in Chapters 4 and 5 are very useful in crisis intervention.

Len who has become disturbed at home

The CPN and her student nurse have six patients to see during the course of the day. Allowing for travelling time, lunch, etc. and the morning's administration, each patient could expect at least half an hour contact time with them. The CPN is also a member of a crisis intervention team covering her area, which means that she may have to interrupt her daily schedule at a moment's notice should the necessity arise.

Halfway through the morning, she receives a call on her radio bleeper. After contacting the health centre she is given the telephone number of a social worker who has been called to a patient's home to deal with a potentially difficult domestic crisis. She rings the social worker who, because he is in the patient's home, is unable to tell her everything on the telephone. However, he does tell her that it is one of her ex-patients, Len, who is experiencing difficulties on a personal level which have generated an abnormal psychological response in him. The CPN is a little unsure about the vagueness of this message but realises that her presence is required. She asks the student to visit the next patient on her list, detailing the purpose of the visit and the method by which the care objectives for the patient should be evaluated. They agree to meet up again later and she then goes to help the social worker.

HISTORY

Crisis Intervention Team is a group of health professionals including psychiatrists, psychologists and social workers as well as nurses who respond to calls for help in dealing with psychiatric problems in the individual's home situation. By working as a team, they bring different skills to bear in resolving the crisis.

At the patient's home

On arrival, the CPN is ushered into the lounge by Len's wife. Len is sitting on the settee with a tearful expression on his face, and adopting a body posture signifying helplessness. The social worker suggests that Len outline what has happened so that the information the CPN needs to help in the crisis situation does not come solely from another 'clinician'. As Len details the circumstances from his point of view, both his wife and the social worker add pieces here and there to give an overall picture of the events leading up to and including the current crisis.

Body posture is the adoption of various poses which may signify to others the mood of the individual. Very often this unspoken method of communication tells you more about people than what they actually say verbally.

Explanatory note: in such a situation, it would be very easy for the social worker to update the CPN by doing all the talking himself. However, it would mean that the information would be mostly secondhand; it might be clouded by his own opinion of the nature of events, and also it would be as an observer, not as the involved individual.

More importantly, it would preclude Len from taking part in the hand over of information, thus denying him the opportunity to take part in the assessment of his own situation. By allowing him to tell the CPN directly what has happened, a more rounded picture can be gained as the other interested parties add their side of the story. In addition, the element of formality that the social worker might bring to the situation is reduced, allowing for a much more relaxed interchange. Finally it offers the social worker an opportunity to take stock of what has happened to date, allowing him to make decisions about his next move.

The CPN discovers the following basic facts:

1 Len's wife has told him that she no longer wishes to share his home.
2 This is not the first time she has threatened to leave, but this time she seriously intends to go.
3 His wife states that she is fed up with his apparent helplessness, lack of drive, self pity and boring outlook on life.

4 Len says he has developed pains in his chest, inability to focus his eyes and general weakness throughout his whole body.

5 Len actually states that he wants to be admitted to hospital because this will convince his wife that there really is something wrong with him.

6 His wife doesn't seem able to bear her husband even touching her hand, let alone showing feeling or emotion towards her.

7 Len presents a picture of a helpless, rejected man.

8 The social worker has been here for an hour and has managed to achieve very little except to clarify for himself what is happening.

9 The situation has got to the point where it is simply becoming repetitive.

It is necessary whilst the CPN makes this appraisal of the situation that she decides in her own mind her next move. She has to show that she has something positive to offer otherwise Len and, more especially his wife, will disregard any input she tries to make. In fact, should she present as being indecisive or hesitant, she may well have a detrimental effect on the whole proceedings, resulting in the wife walking out there and then.

Phase One Development

The CPN decides to establish the background to the current situation, without going over the ground that has already been covered. In particular, with reference to Len's previous history, she wants to know when he started using his current regressive behaviour and how long it has been since his wife developed such negative feelings for him. This is particularly relevant because three years ago Len was discharged from hospital following a depress-

NURSING CARE

Regressive behaviour is the use of behaviour which is more appropriate to an earlier stage in an individual's psychological development.

ive illness and at that time, the CPN had noted quite a strong bond between the husband and wife, totally the opposite to what was present now. Such a change is regarded as being very significant.

Development of Len's current behaviour

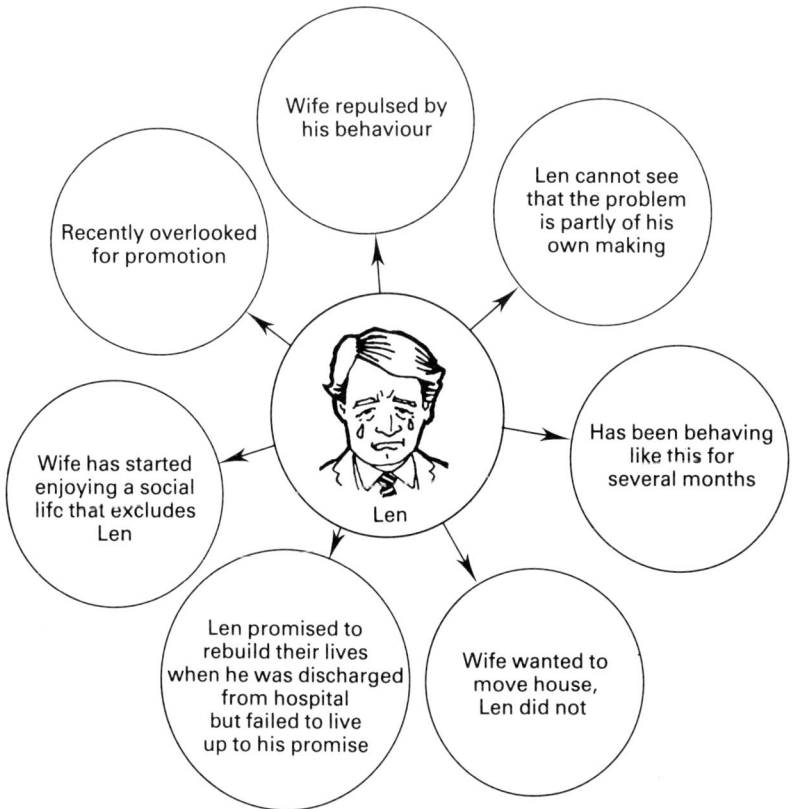

Phase Two Development

Having established the way in which the situation has developed and some of the factors that may have contributed towards it, the next step is to establish the necessity for Len to behave in the way that he does. The CPN notes that his wife becomes verbally abusive towards him when he weeps, saying quite hurtful things about his ability to perform as a man and to live up to her expectation of a husband. Using the skills of active listening and counselling, the CPN discovers the following information:

1 Len actually says that there is nothing wrong with him, though he does admit that he cries a great deal and feels physically weak.
2 He admits there is probably nothing physically wrong with him and therefore his feelings of weakness might stem from somewhere else.
3 He thinks his wife will stay with him if she feels sorry for him.
4 His wife thinks the whole situation is ridiculous and that contrary to what Len believes, it is his helplessness that makes her more determined to leave, not stay.

Although Len appears helpless, he tends at times to lean over to his wife in an attempt to touch her. In doing so, he provokes a hostile response from her. This invasion of her intimate space is, in fact, quite an aggressive thing to do because it is totally inappropriate under these circumstances.

Intimate space is that area around the individual, up to 18 inches, which is reserved for maximum interpersonal stimulation. Entry into this space against the individual's wishes will often provoke discomfort and represent a threat to their personal safety.

Explanatory note: though four types of space have been identified as surrounding the individual, intimate space, personal space, social-consultative space, and public space (Hall 1959), only the intimate and personal ones are significant in this situation. Between husband and wife it would be expected that entry into each other's intimate or personal space would be by tacit agreement. If that agreement is not forthcoming from either one or both parties, it signifies the desire to preclude them from intimacy. If one partner becomes assertive and maintains a comfortable distance between him or herself and the other partner, and the other partner is aware of this fact, any future invasion of space must be considered as a possible, direct attempt at being aggressive. In Len's case, he is pretending to be helpless on one hand yet acting aggressively on the other. His unwillingness to co-operate with his wife might also be considered aggressive, especially if it is within his power to do so. It must also be said that her intolerance of him might be seen as a passively aggressive action. Just which one of them actually started the whole process will probably never be discovered, but it is important that the CPN and the social worker consider the behaviour as it is now, and the relationship that has developed as a consequence of it.

The CPN asks Len why he tries to touch his wife, and he says it is because he loves her. When asked if he realises that it disturbs her, he says that he does but cannot understand why. When asked if he ought not to do it if it upsets her, he says 'yes', and agrees not to do so for the time being.

The CPN then asks his wife why being touched by her husband causes irritation, and she says because she doesn't want him to. After a little discussion, she admits that it is because she is angry with him.

NURSING CARE

Phase Three Development

The next step for the CPN is to help Len and his wife establish the true nature of their feelings about each other. Already the wife has admitted that her anger for Len is the main reason for her own behaviour and not, as she said originally, his feelings as a man. For Len's part, he has begun to admit that he irritates his wife as a subtle means of getting his own back at her.

Identifying the feelings that Len and his wife have about each other

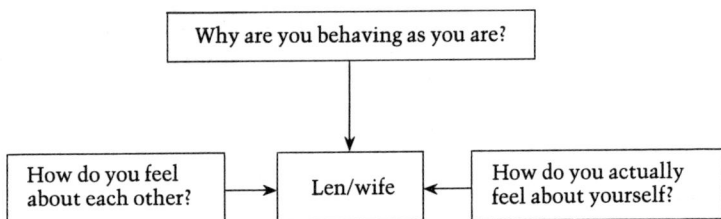

```
                    ┌──────────────────────────────┐
                    │  Why are you behaving as you  │
                    │             are?              │
                    └──────────────┬───────────────┘
                                   │
                                   ▼
┌──────────────────┐     ┌──────────────────┐     ┌──────────────────┐
│  How do you feel │ ──▶ │    Len/wife      │ ◀── │  How do you      │
│  about each      │     │                  │     │  actually        │
│  other?          │     │                  │     │  feel about      │
│                  │     │                  │     │  yourself?       │
└──────────────────┘     └──────────────────┘     └──────────────────┘
```

Although the CPN is mostly concerned with Len's behaviour because he is requesting admission to hospital for it and because it is very maladaptive, the wife must be involved in the reconciliation process otherwise she will fail to see its significance for herself. It will be pointless helping Len to overcome this crisis, if his wife fails to respond in a reciprocal fashion.

Phase Four Development

NURSING CARE

Self abuse is harming oneself in some way, either as an attempt at suicide, a suicidal gesture or some form of self mutilation.

Having established the behavioural problems, and their effects upon each other, the CPN asks Len to identify how his current behaviour of feigned helplessness, threats of self abuse and apparent emotional instability differs from the way he ought to be behaving if he really wants his wife to stay at home. She suggests the possibility that, if he is admitted to hospital, far from keeping his wife he stands a serious threat of losing her. As such, it is in his best interests to remain within the family home and try to develop a method of overcoming their differences.

The two agree to discuss ways by which they can help the other recognise the need for change and to consider the type of behaviour they should adopt to meet that change. His wife is reluctant to remain in the house but eventually agrees to do so for the next 24 hours on the basis of trying to sort out their differences, as agreed between them and the CPN. The CPN agrees to visit at the same time next day to establish progress and help decide what to do next.

<table>
<tr><td>

NURSING
CARE

</td><td>

Evaluation and Follow-up

Two objectives were essential in Len's situation:

</td></tr>
</table>

1   That both he and his wife be involved in coping with the crisis, so that they become aware of the need for change.
2   To ensure that Len did not harm himself in any way while remaining at home, i.e. without being admitted to hospital.

These objectives had been achieved for now and the social worker and CPN discussed them in detail back at the health centre. It was agreed not to stop actively encouraging Len to consider his own behaviour in relation to that of his wife's expectations of him. It was also agreed that, for the next few days, the social worker or the CPN would visit alternately, but would brief each other concerning the visits. Len was to be allowed to solve the problems he faced in his own way as long as it did not develop into a maladaptive way. Finally, it was agreed that the crisis was over for the time being because Len and his wife were talking to each other again, he was no longer demanding hospital admission, and he did not currently intend self abuse.

The crisis intervention team would discuss Len's care at the next meeting to establish if the approach adopted by the CPN had been successful or not, to learn from it if it had been, and try to decide how it could have been improved if not.

Len and his wife split up three months later

despite counselling from the CPN. Len did not abuse himself in any way and through counselling was able to maintain himself independently in the community without the disruptive necessity of a hospital admission.

<table>
<tr><td>

**TEST
YOURSELF**

</td><td>

1 Identify the various phases that might be used to bring a crisis to a satisfactory conclusion.
2 In the care study, why was it necessary to involve both Len and his wife in the intervention?
3 What techniques can the nurse use in a crisis situation to collect enough immediate information to be able to direct the discussion in a positive way?
4 Why was it important for Len and his wife to try to resolve their difficulties at home rather than having Len admitted to a psychiatric unit because of his behaviour?

</td></tr>
</table>

<table>
<tr><td>

**FURTHER
READING**

</td><td>

BUTTERWORTH, C. & SKIDMORE, D. 1981. *Caring for the mentally ill in the community.* London: Croom Helm.
HALL, E. 1959. *The silent language.* New York: Doubleday & Co.
MURGATROYD, S. & WOOLFE, R. 1982. *Coping with stress.* London: Harper-Row.
MURGATROYD, S. & WOOLFE, R. 1985. *Helping families in distress.* London: Harper-Row.

</td></tr>
</table>

8 The Use of Social Skills Therapy

Interpersonal
behaviour is the
behaviour we use
in our contact with
other people,
including the
things we say and
the things we do.

In recent years the study of interpersonal behaviour has emerged as a significant area of work trying to help people who appear to have difficulties in their ability to communicate with others. Indeed some specialists have made the point that interpersonal difficulties may be the cause of what we term 'mental disorder', whilst others have put forward the theory that 'mental disorder' *causes* interpersonal problems. This in no way denies the possibility that the person may be mentally *ill*. However, it tends to place the emphasis on the observable behaviour performed by the individual and witnessed by others as being indicative that the person is not at ease in social contact, and that others may not be at ease with him.

In particular, those who subscribe to the behavioural approach in psychology have described various features which together amount to the ability to interact in a satisfactory manner. These components of interaction are usually referred to as *social skills*.

What are Social Skills?

Have you ever been lost for words when meeting someone for the first time? What do you say? It sometimes seems the more you try to make informal introductory conversation, the more difficult and embarrassing the situation becomes. You become anxious and self conscious, and the other person responds by looking bored and eventually moving away to someone else with whom he feels more comfortable. Conversely, some people seem to possess a magnetism which holds people spellbound and words just flow with effortless ease.

How can people be so different? In truth, most people seem to experience both situations at various points in social contact and much depends on how they feel at the time. However, certain factors make social interaction more comfortable and rewarding, and it is the skilled use of those factors which can determine the response we receive from other people.

It is important to look at the person with whom you are talking in a way which shows genuine concern and interest. We do this by eye to eye contact and by facial expression, and we try to avoid yawning or looking past the person at the clock on the wall. Frequent eye contact and the gestures of smiling and nodding are methods by which we can show the other person we are interested in them and in what they are saying.

We all seem to have an area around us which is only for ourselves (and invited guests!) and respect for this social distance is vital in interactions. If we invade someone else's private area, then we are likely to be repelled because of the discomfort it causes. Standing or sitting at the right distance from the other person avoids posing a threat of invasion and allows each person to concentrate on making social rather than physical contact.

Not everything we say is expressed in the words we speak and we convey as many ideas by gestures as we do by verbal language. Indeed it is often more difficult to control our non-verbal messages than our verbal ones and if the two do not synchronise we can cause confusion to others, and to ourselves. Certain gestures are appropriate for particular situations.

Social distance In this particular sense we are talking about a physical space rather than the way a sociologist might refer to a feeling of alienation from classes of people in society.

Non-verbal is any form of behaviour which does not involve the spoken word but which may include tone of voice.

For example, pictures of Sir Winston Churchill with two fingers raised can convey a very different message than might be intended by an angry soccer player making a gesture to the referee.

Speaking clearly, at the right volume and speed is important in social interaction; if we mumble or shout we are likely to find difficulty in making contact with other people. Picture then the person who stands too close to you and avoids eye contact whilst mumbling under his breath and blushing furiously. How do you respond? It is just possible you may think the person is mentally unwell. Social skills therapy attempts to help people, who have lost or never developed these skills, to learn and practise them in order that they may become effective, successful communicators.

Social skills components

Non-verbal	Verbal
Facial expression	Saying what you feel
Gestures	Asking appropriate questions
Eye contact	Making relevant comments
Posture	Telling others what you want
Spatial awareness	
Tone of voice	
Body contact	

Social Skills Training and the CPN

It has been said that psychiatric and mental handicap nurses derive more benefit from experience in social skills than in being sent for eight weeks to a general hospital during basic training (Carr *et al.* 1980). Certainly the whole field of social skills therapy is a fertile one for the CPN, who is in a good position to help unskilled people develop within this vital area of interpersonal communication.

The close relationship between the community nurse and the client can be the foundation of successful social skills training, either on a one to one basis in the client's home or with a group in a room at the local health centre. Away from the clinical confines of a hospital the client can learn and practise social skills in the setting to which they are appropriate.

What form can social skills therapy take? The first move might be to assess the client's problems in interpersonal communication by allowing him to make a self evaluation of his problems (and his assets). This can be achieved by pencil and paper type tests such as 'brainstorming' in which the client is asked to write anything which enters his mind after being given a topic, or by 'sentence completion' tests, as in the examples below:

1 People make me feel ....
2 I hate ....
3 My worst fear is ....

When this problem identification process is complete, the nurse and the client can set together objectives which will lead to the development of behaviour that is more successful and more satisfying.

Learning strategies in social skills training (after Trower
et al. 1978)

1	Demonstration	Modelling the skill in a simple way for the client to observe
2	Imitation	Client role-plays the skill he has seen the trainer demonstrate
3	Feedback	Receive praise in a way that the client sees as rewarding
4	Practice	Following feedback the client practises points which may have proved to be particularly difficult for him and receives encouragement from the trainer
5	Homework	The application of what has been learned to the real situation and reporting back on success/failure

Having set the objectives, methods of learning can be used to develop and reinforce the skills necessary for success. Various learning strategies can be used and these will be expanded as an actual example in the case study which forms the second part of this chapter.

Learning depends on knowing just what is to be learned, why it is to be learned, and how it is to be learned. The technique of giving positive reward for developing toward the ultimate objective is central to social skills training. The reward need not necessarily be in a material form since the development of successful social interaction often serves as reward in itself. Praise and recognition of success go a long way to reinforcing learning.

The training routine can follow the pattern outlined by Trower *et al.* (1978), as does our care study example:

1   Decide upon and arrange the setting in which training will take place.
2   Revise the previous session (if any).
3   Develop and teach a single skill with a description of its function, components and instructions for use.
4   A learning routine of demonstration, imitation, feedback, practice and guidance.
5   Homework assignments on the training sessions.

George who has left the long stay hospital

George is 53 years old and has been an in-patient in various psychiatric hospitals for the past 15 years. As you might imagine, after such a long period of time in an institutional environment he has developed a type of behaviour which is appropriate only to that setting. As a consequence of this, when discharged after a long and carefully planned rehabilitation programme, it was increasingly difficult to participate fully in the new community situation that he found himself in. Living now as he did in a house with three other ex-patients, he found it easier to relapse into his old institutional behaviour during the evenings and at weekends, rather than try to behave in a manner more appropriate to an independent and self supporting individual.

Institutional behaviour. Living for even a short while in a relatively restricted (socially) environment can lead to behaviour which is acceptable in that situation, but not in the community at large.

Sister Susan Gray, George's community psychiatric nurse, had met with him many times before he was discharged from hospital. She had monitored his progress in the rehabilitation programme which had concentrated on social and life skills. Together they had discussed those areas with which he had found difficulty. She had worked with the hospital-based team of nurses, occupational therapists and psychologists to try and make the programme as realistic as possible. She knew that George could perform well in a group setting with people he knew well and trusted, and that he was able to participate in a considerable amount of personal life skills activities reasonably well. However, she was aware that certain deficiencies in his contact skills were reducing

George's skill rating on discharge

Life skill	Not competent				Competent
	1	2	3	4	5
1 Personal hygiene					√
2 Dressing/Selection of clothing					√
3 Housekeeping/Cleaning, etc.				√	
4 Cooking				√	
5 Management of finance					√
6 Use of public transport			√		
7 Shopping		√			
8 Contact with newcomers		√			
9 Recreational activities			√		
10 Involvement in community facilities		√			
11 Employment capability				√	
12 Problem solving			√		

his personal effectiveness and the hospital situation was an unreal environment in which to redress the balance.

During George's last few weeks on the hostel ward prior to his discharge, he and Susan discussed ways in which she would be able to help him overcome some of his difficulties. She outlined the relationship that would develop between them, indicating that at first she would be visiting him quite regularly to monitor his progress and assess his ability to function on his own. As the pattern of his life unfolded, a reappraisal of her role would be made, but at all times he would take part in the decision-making that determined her level of commitment to him. It was also agreed that the problem areas identified in George's skill ability before discharge would be considered in more detail once they had been put to the test in a more practical and realistic environment.

Susan's main concern at first was to get George settled into his new environment as easily as possible so that he felt comfortable and safe. That achieved, she then had to consider the problems he faced with certain areas of his social skills, namely those which centred around meeting people, often for the first time.

Problem Identification

NURSING
CARE

George and Susan sat in the lounge of the residence and talked about the skills rating chart. George was already aware of his difficulties with meeting people and despite several attempts at overcoming them whilst an inpatient, he had never felt confident enough to really tackle them with any purpose. The main problem had been that he did not really have the motivation to succeed because he knew that he had a safe haven in the hospital, and as this aspect of his rehabilitation programme did not carry quite as much weight as some of the more practical skills of living, his discharge would still come through even without success in this area. The other main difficulty was that these contact skills actually generated far more anxiety for him than any of the others and he felt it was far more acceptable to avoid them if he possibly could. As a consequence of this, they had become even more difficult to tackle because of the fact that he kept putting them off.

Explanatory note: George's problem here is not dissimilar to those encountered by many of us. Often we are faced with difficult tasks which we put off because of their difficulty, always telling ourselves that we are simply waiting for a more convenient time to do them. In effect we are postponing possible failure – always something awkward for anyone to deal with. The more we put the job off, the more unpleasant it becomes, and the more difficult it seems. Eventually it assumes horrific proportions, totally out of context with the original trouble. Sometimes we avoid doing the job altogether; on other occasions something exceptional happens which forces us into making a more positive decision and we tackle the job. Often as not we discover it to be a far less harrowing task than we originally envisaged because, in truth, we are far more clever than we give ourselves credit for. Afterwards we wonder why on earth we had so much difficulty. In George's case, the situation is slightly different in that he has so little personal confidence in his own abilities that it is extremely difficult to be positive about the eventual outcome of his attempt at social contact.

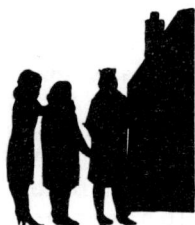

Between them, George and Susan decide that the best way to tackle the immediate problem would be to link several areas of difficulty together and construct one set of problems. They isolate the shopping and social contact areas as one and the same problem because they both give rise to the same feelings of stress and anxiety that inhibit George's ability to perform effectively.

Skills Objectives

Next they decide upon a series of objectives that George might realistically hope to achieve. Susan takes into consideration his current level of performance which she knows to be very poor. His skills rating in both areas is quite low but there is an indication that he is capable of some activity. They discuss just what he can do at present, and the feelings and difficulties that he faces when confronted with this problem. George has not had to shop for himself for a considerably long period of time but here in the residence he will have to assume responsibility for these aspects of home management with his fellow residents and he has to perform this job well.

The objectives are set in a sequence. The first objective is to simply go to a shop and ask for one pre-selected item, preferably in a self-service area or somewhere where little actual contact will be necessary. The next objective will either increase the number of items or the amount of contact. Eventual objectives will involve much more complex tasks, but it may be many months before they are achieved. Each objective has to be successfully achieved before the next can be attempted. A time limit is set for their evaluation. George will ultimately set this time limit himself because he must pace himself with the requirements of each task. He will not be rushed or hurried into achieving objectives and only when he is satisfied with his own performance will he be expected to progress to the next. Support, guidance and reassurance will be necessary all the time and Susan has to plan her visits to George to coincide with those times she feels she is most likely to be of assistance to him. This might be initially whilst he attempts to achieve his objectives and later on at the time he evaluates his activities.

Methodology

They discuss several different approaches to dealing with the problem, although it is agreed that initially George must attempt to buy something from the local foodstore whilst Susan observes him so that she can gain some idea of his current ability. The following alternatives are then open to George:

Modelling is
presenting an
example of
behaviour which
represents a
standard to be
achieved.

1 Susan completes the same task as George whilst he observes her performance so that he can model his next attempt on her. Such modelling techniques could also be used to increase other elements of his social contact skills.

2 George could go shopping with one of the other residents to observe how he goes about tackling the same problem. After comparing the performance of Susan and of his fellow resident, he might be able to select a style or approach that would suit himself and not be totally dependent on imitating the skills of others.

3 He could be allowed to select different types of shops to go into to see which ones generate the most or least stress.

4 He could enact his speech and approach to shop keepers in a role play situation in the residence, either using Susan or other residents to play the part of the shopkeeper. In this way he could rehearse those opening gambits and sentences used readily by others without thinking about them.

5 He could vary the items he needed to buy.

6 He could visit small shops in the company of Susan and meet the proprietor, explain his difficulty and with her help find out a little about the people he might encounter in the shop.

7 He could walk around shops to identify where things were so that he felt more familiar

with the surroundings. Hopefully this might boost his confidence a little so that when he actually had to purchase something he felt better able to do so, thus giving himself a more positive approach to the problem.

They constructed a contract that George would comply with. Basically this was a document that would serve two purposes:

1 It would identify for George what areas of difficulty he had, what he was expected to do to be able to counteract them and how he was to go about it. It would also remind him of his achievements to date, but most importantly it would provide him with a target to aim for. Hopefully this would generate the motivation necessary for him to begin the actual process of regaining his social contact skills.

2 It would provide Susan with a written record of George's progress and a baseline from which to make evaluations for future objectives.

George's initial skills contract

Skill problem	Objective	Approach
I don't know how to speak to people when I go into shops to buy things	I can buy one item from a selected shop	1 I will select one item to buy
		2 I will say 'Good morning' to the shop assistant
		3 I will tender the right money
		4 I will say 'thank you and goodbye' to the assistant
		5 When speaking I will look at the assistant and not stare at the ground
		6 I will speak with a clear voice so that the assistant is easily able to hear me

Progress

Over a period of 12 weeks, George tackled the problem of social contact in a shopping situation. Each week he set himself a different objective, each objective more exacting than the last and each requiring him to do a little more each time. Initially, Susan accompanied him to the local shops, encouraging him and helping him decide upon the people he would approach. He shopped once each day and after each attempt would re-enact his performance with her back at the residence. Both good and bad points were identified so that they could either be used again or avoided in the future. Gradually George's level of performance increased and he was able to approach his responsibilities within the residence reasonably successfully. The actual process of shopping did not really present him with too much difficulty because many of the items he had to purchase were already identified by either necessity or by the other residents. His contact with several of the local shopkeepers, although not perfect, became much more acceptable, especially as they began to get to know him and greeted him accordingly.

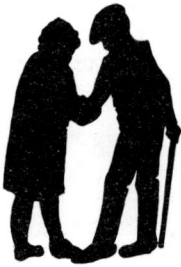

In many ways, this success defeated the object of the exercise because it meant that George was no longer making contact with people he did not know. However, it meant that through the secondary medium of shopping, he had made the first steps in increasing his ability to cope with the pressure placed upon him in the area of social contact.

Evaluation

After each week's objective, either successful or not, both George and Susan reflected upon the week's activities. Susan needed to establish whether or not George was able to progress to the next objective, and if her own input was providing sufficient support and guidance. She also needed to decide upon new strategies if possible so that the whole process was interesting and creative for George.

George needed to establish for himself that he really was making progress, and to see just how he was achieving it. In this way he would be in a better position to reproduce the skills he was learning in new and more challenging situations.

Susan identified the successful completion of initial skills activity as having several 'spin off' repercussions for George's progress in the community:

1 It gave him more confidence in himself.
2 It gave him positive feelings about himself.
3 It promoted problem solving skills.
4 It generated belief in his own abilities.
5 It provided a spring board for him to increase his contact skills.

As a result of this, Susan was able to discuss with George new areas for him to tackle using the skills he had acquired whilst learning to shop successfully. She had combined a simple living skill, that of shopping, with a far more complex one of contact with others, to provide an interesting and purposeful way of increasing George's personal effectiveness as an individual. She would continue to support and guide him, allowing him to set his own pace of progress, and eventually teaching him to set his own goals. Her contact with him would gradually decrease as necessary, though she would always be on hand to help him when he needed her. She must show tolerance and understanding of his situation and an acceptance of his possible limitations. As he constructed a problem solving network to help him deal with situations as they arose, she would monitor their effects, guiding where necessary, but often simply providing encouragement. George might never regain total comprehension in the area of social contact but he, at least, would never be frustrated by his own inabilities to get what he needed through social interaction.

TEST YOURSELF

1 Identify the main problem areas George experienced because of his long period of hospitalisation.
2 What were the main procedural steps in the teaching of George's contact skills?
3 Make a note of the method you use to make yourself feel at ease with people you meet for the very first time.
4 If you are working in the community and face the same problems that Susan had, how might your knowledge of your own contact skills help you guide a patient in the production of his own skills programme?

FURTHER READING

ARGYLE, M. 1983. *The Psychology of Interpersonal Behaviour*. Harmondsworth: Penguin.
BERNE, E. 1984. *What do you say after you say hello?* London: Corgi.
BERNE, E. 1985. *Games People Play*. Harmondsworth: Penguin.
CARR, P. J., BUTTERWORTH, C. A. & HODGES, B. E. 1979. *Community Psychiatric Nursing*. Edinburgh: Churchill Livingstone.
PRIESTLEY, P., MCQUIRE, J., FLEGG, D., HEMSLEY, V. & WELHAM, D. 1978. *Social Skills and Personal Problem Solving*. London: Tavistock.
TROWER, P., BRYANT, B. & ARGYLE, M. 1978. *Social Skills and Mental Health*. London: Methuen.

9 The Future of Community Psychiatric Nursing

As stated previously, the psychiatric nurse working full time in the community is a relatively recent concept. The last few years have seen increasing numbers of CPNs and this growth is expected not only to continue but to gain momentum as community care policies develop throughout health regions (CPNA Survey 1985). The emergence of the CPN as a practitioner who is distinguishable from the traditional hospital nurse has highlighted the need for careful consideration to be given to the future in terms of service provision and professional development. The training and education of CPNs coupled with a clear policy for providing community psychiatric nursing must be the two-pronged approach to development.

Education

Currently the psychiatric nursing student in basic training spends as little as 8 per cent of learning time in the community allocation. This implies that even a Registered Mental Nurse, recently qualified, can gain only some appreciation of the complexities of community psychiatric nursing rather than a background which would enable competent practice without further education. The question, therefore, is what form that further education should take and how it should be facilitated in a practical, economic way available to those who are currently practising and future CPNs.

Currently the National Boards for Nursing and Midwifery are responsible for post-registration nurse education. The English National Board provides a course for community psychiatric nursing (ENB course number 811) which is full time and lasts for 42 weeks, including practical experience and theoretical input. The course is offered by schools of nursing and by colleges of technical and further education. In the 1985 CPNA National Survey Update, it was discovered that only 22.4 per cent of the CPN workforce had completed the course and, therefore, the need for further education is great amongst already practising CPNs, let alone those who are still joining the expanding service. The need is for more courses to be established and for funding to be made available in order that the backlog of 'undertrained' CPNs can be reduced. Little research has been carried out to confirm the effectiveness of these courses, but CPNs themselves firmly support the notion of further training and the Community Psychiatric Nurses' Association appears to be in favour of making the qualification mandatory for practice. The courses currently available do not appear to be capable of providing enough places to make such a notion reality, but at the same time areas of excellence in the education of CPNs are emerging and a distinct body of knowledge is developing which can be the springboard for the professional development of the CPN and the enhancement of the service provided.

Explanatory note: during your community allocation, you should look carefully at the way a CPN's work differs from that of a hospital nurse, and try to identify what skills, knowledge and attitudes you think should be developed in order to practise in a competent way.

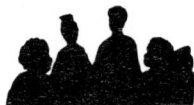

Professional Development

Currently the definition of the role of the CPN is the basis of much debate and although some investigations have identified important functions, it is still difficult to state this role in a way which is nationally accepted. This state of affairs is not a poor reflection on the CPN service generally, but merely a common experience for an emerging specialty and the debate is lively, constructive and showing signs of reaching consensus. Good work is taking place particularly within the Community Psychiatric Nurses' Association, and the forum offered by those establishments providing the course for CPNs.

Research into practice is essential in any profession and should always provide the pointer for the future. The ideas as to professional development are centred around a number of questions which should also be of concern to you during your community allocation. We suggest that in an attempt to gain a greater understanding of your own clinical experience during your community allocation, you look for the answers to the following questions:

1   Should the CPN be a specialist within a particular area of skills or a general practitioner of psychiatric nursing?
2   Where is the best place to base a CPN? (e.g. hospital, health centre, etc.)
3   How accountable is the CPN in terms of personal and professional responsibilities?
4   How does the development of the nursing process apply to the practice of psychiatric nursing in the community?
5   What research evidence can you find as to the effectiveness and quality of community psychiatric nursing?
6   Should the CPN develop toward true primary care and health education?

Conclusion

The experience of community psychiatric nursing is exciting, interesting and crammed with opportunities for learning. The transition from hospital to community care for the mentally disordered is a continuous process and it offers the opportunity for the nurse to develop skills which otherwise may have never emerged under other circumstances. This, in many ways, must account for the high level of motivation and professional commitment you will encounter among CPNs during your experience with them. A positive but critical approach to your experience will enable you to make a contribution to the most significant area of change in psychiatric nursing to be seen in recent years.

FURTHER READING

C.P.N.A. 1985. *The Clinical Responsibilities of the Community Psychiatric Nurse.* London: C.P.N.A.
C.P.N.A. 1985. *The 1985 C.P.N.A. National Survey Update.* London: C.P.N.A.
REED, J. & LOMAS, G. (ed) 1984. *Psychiatric Services in the Community: Developments and Innovations.* Beckenham: Croom Helm.

INDEX